The Incredible Journey

The Emergence of Froedtert Hospital and
Southeastern Wisconsin's Academic Medical Center

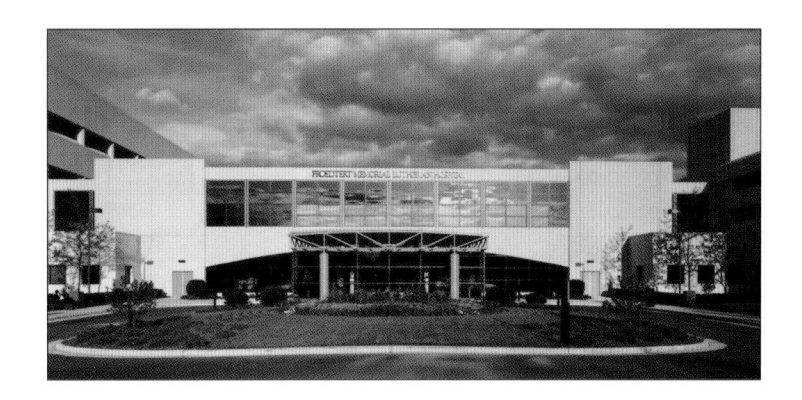

James F. King

Published by

Froedtert HOSPITAL
Froedtert & Community Health
MILWAUKEE, WISCONSIN

The Incredible Journey: The Emergence of Froedtert Hospital and Southeastern Wisconsin's Academic Medical Center by James F. King

Copyright © 2007 by Froedtert Memorial Lutheran Hospital
All rights reserved. Published 2007

All photography in this book (except where noted) is either public domain or the property of Froedtert Hospital and is used with permission.

Editor: Liz Hill
Editorial Consultant: Carolyn Washburn
Design and Typography: Kate Hawley
Index: Carol Roberts
Production Coordinator: Susan Pittelman

ISBN-13: 978-0-9798920-0-4
Library of Congress Control Number: 2007937643

Printed in the United States

Froedtert HOSPITAL
Froedtert & Community Health

9200 West Wisconsin Avenue
Milwaukee, WI 53226
414.805.3000
www.froedtert.com

To my father Joseph M. King, MD

and

the faculty, staff, and patients of Froedtert Hospital

past, present, and future

Contents

Foreword by William D. Petasnick and Dean K. Roe . . . . *vii*
Preface . . . . *ix*

Part One   **1857–1959**
Chapter 1	A Fortune Is Born in the Ashes	3
Chapter 2	Beginning the Long Journey	8
Chapter 3	Surveying the Healthcare Landscape	11
Chapter 4	A Trust for the Future	17
Chapter 5	In Pursuit of Funding	21

Part Two   **1960–1969**
Chapter 6	The Stage Is Set	25
Chapter 7	Another Medical Center Site	27
Chapter 8	Froedtert Hospital Corporation Formed	30
Chapter 9	The Greater Milwaukee Committee and the Politicians	34
Chapter 10	Enter the Political Leadership	37
Chapter 11	Help from the Hospital Area Planning Committee	41
Chapter 12	Pursuit of Froedtert's Goal and Purpose	47
Chapter 13	Medical School Faces Crisis	49

Part Three   **1970–1979**
Chapter 14	Into the Turbulent Seventies	55
Chapter 15	The New County Board	57
Chapter 16	Lining Up the Leases	61
Chapter 17	Medical School Signs Lease	70
Chapter 18	One Crisis after Another	73
Chapter 19	Need for a Medical Center?	79
Chapter 20	The Bumpy Road to Approval	81
Chapter 21	All Tied Up	86
Chapter 22	At Last! Groundbreaking	93
Chapter 23	Merger Problems	97
Chapter 24	Problems at County General Hospital	99
Chapter 25	Building a Hospital and a Staff	102

Part Four	**1980–2005**	
Chapter 26	Organizing the Staff	109
Chapter 27	Opening Day!	113
Chapter 28	The Changing Hospital Scene	115
Chapter 29	Troublesome Times Ahead	117
Chapter 30	Changing the Face of Healthcare	122
Chapter 31	Gale-Force Winds of Change Begin a New Era	125
Epilogue	**2006 and Beyond**	137
	And the Whirlwind Continues	139
About the Author		145
Index		147

Foreword

We are thoroughly convinced that the development of a major comprehensive medical center, including a first-rate medical school, is extremely important to the health and well-being of citizens in this area.

Greater Milwaukee Committee, Heil Report, 1965

On September 14, 1977, approximately twelve years after the release of the Heil Report, Froedtert Hospital officials broke ground for what was to become Southeastern Wisconsin's premier academic medical center. Flashing a bright smile, Mary Froedtert, widow of the hospital's benefactor Kurtis R. Froedtert, lifted the first shovel of dirt to officially begin construction of the $41 million facility that was her late husband's dream. Through the assistance and perseverance of community leaders, and through what was to later be deemed as an incredible journey, Kurtis R. Froedtert's dream was to become a reality.

Three years later, on a sunny September afternoon in 1980, Froedtert Hospital opened its doors and another phase of our incredible journey began, moving steadily toward the vision of Kurtis Froedtert.

Today Froedtert Hospital is a major academic acute care medical center that offers the most advanced treatment to patients with complex medical and surgical problems, broadens the frontiers of medical knowledge through clinical research, and trains the next generation of health professionals. In partnership with the Medical College of Wisconsin, it has emerged as one of the few elite academic medical centers in the country.

The year 2005 marked the twenty-fifth anniversary of Froedtert Hospital. As we celebrated our past and looked toward the future, we felt that it would be important to document the story of Kurtis R. Froedtert's vision to build a hospital for a city he loved. We asked Jim King to write the story of Froedtert. Jim not only worked at Froedtert Hospital for sixteen years, he also practically grew up on the County Grounds. Jim has done an excellent job of capturing the challenges and the successes of the hospital's history, and we are excited to share this story with you. Please join us as we retrace this incredible journey.

William D. Petasnick *Dean K. Roe*
President and CEO President/CEO Emeritus

Preface

This is a story about Froedtert Memorial Lutheran Hospital and the development of the Milwaukee Regional Medical Center. It is not an archival history replete with footnotes, since the hospital continues to write its role as a preeminent source of patient care, clinical research, and education. This is a story about one man's vision and wish to build a hospital for a city he loved. It is a story of persistence and patience practiced by Froedtert trustees, hospital administration, and board of directors members over a tumultuous span of almost a half century. It is a story of how the elected supervisors and executives of Milwaukee County fulfilled their duties as stewards of the land and institutions to hammer out compromises with private entities to form this medical center.

The pages also contain a salute to four men who, in decades past, pioneered excellent patient care and teaching to establish the foundation upon which this center rests today. And, sadly, these pages relate how the economics of today's competitive healthcare market brought about the decision to close the county hospital after more than a century of service.

This land and its institutions have been part of my family for more than eighty years. My father spent his professional life at County General Hospital caring for the sick and teaching hundreds of young men and women to become compassionate physicians and surgeons. Since there is this historical family connection, I was asked to write the story of the hospital and the medical center when I retired from Froedtert after sixteen years on a staff of great people. It has been a labor of love and has taken far too long to complete.

I am indebted to many people who have given of their time to assist in this work. My special note of gratitude extends to a few people no longer with us but are remembered fondly: County Executives John Doyne and William O'Donnell for enlightenment on the politics of healthcare; Margaret Fuchs, former administrative secretary, for the perfect file of news clippings; and Dan Hurley, auxilian, for assembling and copying historical references.

Providing ongoing contributions to this volume were Dean Roe and Bill Petasnick, past and present Froedtert CEOs, who provided valuable insights on administrative responsibilities in the planning and formation of Froedtert Hospital and the Milwaukee Regional Medical Center and the continued growth of a teaching hospital's mission. Interviews with Jerry Apple; Ralph Andreano, PhD; Michael Bolger, president, Medical College of Wisconsin; Tom Brophy; Attorney Charles Mulcahy; Louis Pascek, PhD; and John Petersen, MD, provided information on key negotiating issues. To Karen LeSage: my deepest gratitude for her well-written story of Froedtert's acquisition of the John Doyne Hospital assets in 1995. She was an integral participant in that most significant event.

Thanks to Liz Hill for editing this wordy tome and to Carolyn Bellin for wielding a soft whip to get this finished. The cementing element to all of this has been Joyce Brunau, whose memory, patience, and detailed filing system answered every question raised about events of the last thirty years. Finally, I send my appreciation and note of thanks to all the Froedtert staff who patiently waited for this to be finished. It is.

James F. King

Part One

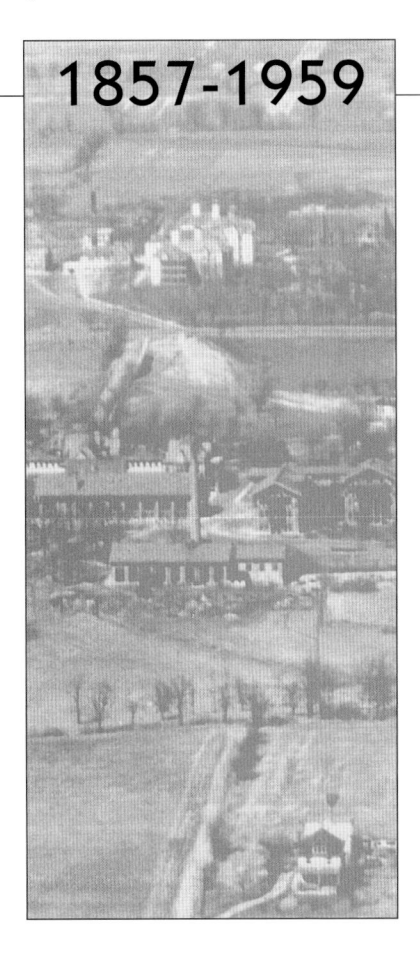

1857-1959

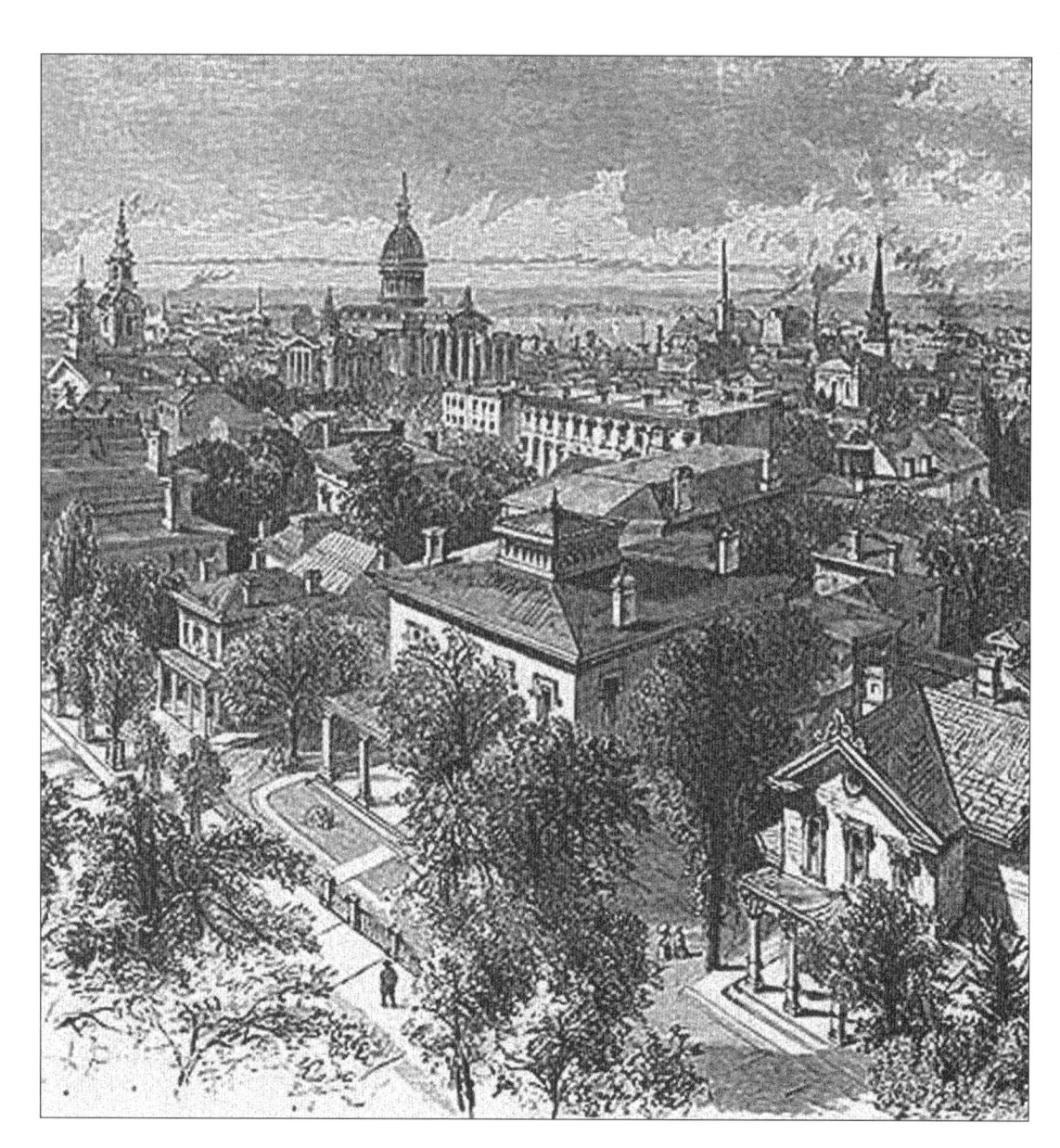

*Milwaukee, Wisconsin,
late 1800s*

Chapter 1

A Fortune Is Born in the Ashes
1857-1951

By the time volunteer firefighters arrived in horse-drawn equipment, the small brewery was engulfed in flames. Despite the volunteers' efforts, flames consumed the Christbaum and Kehrein Brewery at North Fifth and Cherry Streets, just a few blocks north of today's Bradley Center. The once-thriving brewing enterprise was reduced to smoldering embers. It was a fire for the future. Only the brewery's malt house was spared that day in 1857 when Milwaukee was still a fledgling city.

Although a century-and-a-half ago the small brewery lay in ruins, the surviving malt house represented the proverbial phoenix of a new and prosperous enterprise in Milwaukee. Eventually that business generated the fortune used to help build Froedtert Hospital and foster the concept of a major academic medical center for Southeastern Wisconsin.

Today most people are unaware that it took almost fifty years of unforeseen twists and turns, controversy, numerous studies, litigation, rejections, politics, and compromise before Froedtert Hospital became recognized as a major resource for the Milwaukee area. In the end, the establishment of Froedtert Hospital and the development of this major medical center reflect the classic example of private and public sectors working for the good of a community.

Underscoring the nearly three decades of planning and recurring setbacks was a level of persistence by Froedtert Hospital trustees and community leaders to achieve a goal that would best implement the wishes of Kurtis R. Froedtert. This Milwaukee industrialist and philanthropist sought to build a hospital in his name to serve the community he loved so well. While the terms of his will did not declare that the hospital be a major teaching, research, and patient care facility in a medical center setting, the Froedtert Hospital Trust was the seed from which this medical center flowered.

Since the mid-nineteenth century, the Froedtert name has been a part of Milwaukee's history when the city became a magnet for the many skilled craftsmen from Europe. German immigration played a major role in setting the economic tone and strength of Milwaukee in its earliest years. The city teemed with German immigrants skilled in the printing trades,

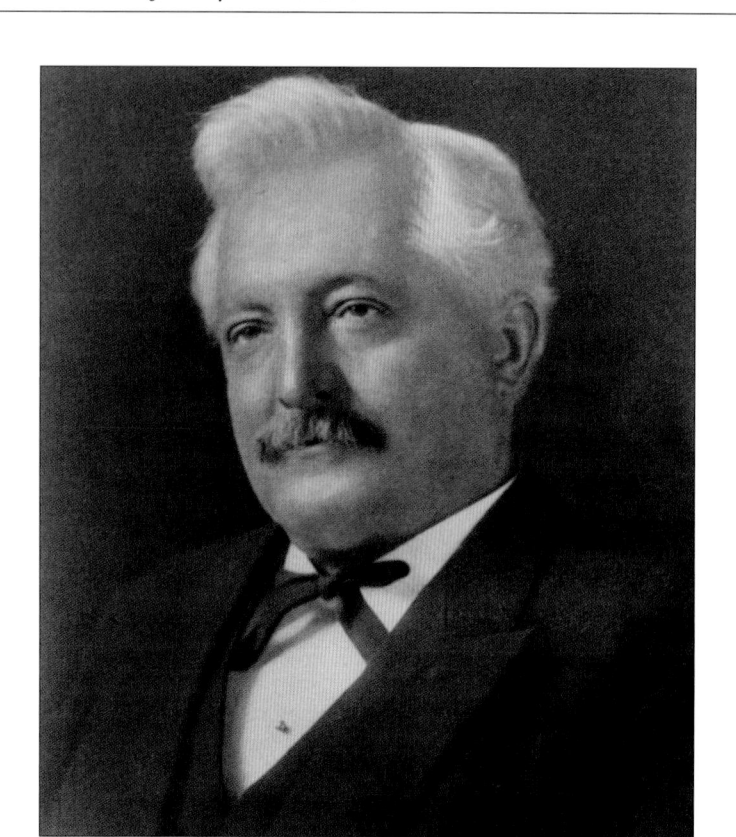

Kurtis Froedtert's father, William

tool-and-die making, baking, millwork, and cabinetry. It was the immigrant *braumeisters*—brew masters—from Germany whose knowledge of the art of brewing beer forged a significant role as an economic force in the city's history. While heavy industry was said to be the muscle of Milwaukee's early economy, it was the brewing artistry that added the grace to the city's bustling economy and gained world acclaim for Milwaukee as the nation's beer capital.

William and Jacob Froedtert were among the industrious German stock who settled in the Midwest grain belt. They had left their birthplace at Nordheim, Hessen Kasel, Germany, and followed the migration to America and the Midwest. For the two brothers, an apprenticeship in the flour, seed, and feed business in Germany presaged the formation of the Froedtert Brothers Commission Company in Milwaukee. Following the brewery fire in 1857, the unscathed malt house represented a business opportunity that the Froedtert brothers seized. They bought the malt house and incorporated as the Froedtert Grain and Malting Company.

As the brewing industry grew, so did the malt business, because a bushel of malt was needed for each barrel of beer. As principal suppliers of this key beer ingredient, the Froedtert Grain and Malting Company experienced steady growth, providing the malt for Milwaukee breweries and other breweries throughout the Midwest.

While breweries were the Froedtert brothers' major customers, they had others. Many German immigrants drank a roasted barley beverage because coffee was uncommon in Europe. Malt was also sold to laboratories and pharmaceutical firms and was used for the manufacture of certain liquors, malt syrup, breakfast foods, and concentrates.

Kurtis R. Froedtert was born on June 3, 1887, the son of William Froedtert. It has been said that Kurtis Froedtert always had an interest in science, especially medicine, but strong family ties and his father's death would put Kurt Froedtert at the helm of the Froedtert Grain and Malting

Company. At seventeen, he graduated from the old German English Academy, now known as Milwaukee University School. As a teenager, he spent summers shoveling grain into bags at the Froedtert plant. He went on to Orchard Lake Military Academy, near Detroit, where he was the class valedictorian. He was offered three Ivy League scholarships. The young Kurt planned to go on to college to study medicine, but his father had other ideas. He enrolled his son in the Hantke Brewing School in Detroit. Kurt returned to Milwaukee to begin a career in the malting world under the guidance of his father. His interest in medicine and other sciences never waned. In later years, his grasp of the technical problems of his many enterprises was sure and swift.

The course was firmly set for Kurt Froedtert when his father died in 1915. The twenty-eight-year-old assumed the reins of the company and began an era of remarkable growth for the Froedtert Grain and Malting Company. His first major business move was significant, bold, and highly successful, as were many other ventures throughout his business career. Two years after his father's death, Kurt learned of trouble at a competing malt company. He bought the plant in Winona, Minnesota, with $240,000 in borrowed funds. Additional acquisitions pushed Froedtert malt production to about 250,000 bushels of malt a year. Some thirty-five years later, at the time of Kurt's death in 1951, annual malt production reached 22 million bushels. Froedtert Grain and Malting Company was the largest malting company in the world.

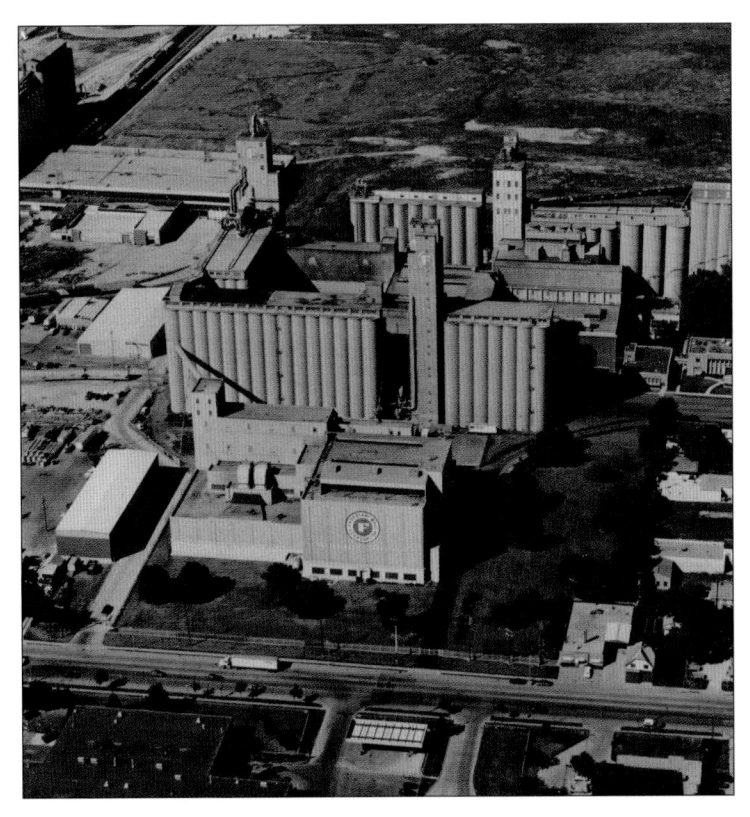

In a feature article in the *Milwaukee Journal* in January 1955, reporter Walter Monfried wrote of the immense energy that Froedtert threw into his labors:

> He sought to know, personally, all the brew masters in the country. He was their friend. If they had difficulties, or needed jobs, he did his best to solve their troubles, and frequently did. If a brewer's product turned out flat or otherwise unsatisfactory, Froedtert would take off two or three days and make the long journey to help his customer.

Froedtert Grain and Malting Company

Monfried quoted Froedtert as saying, somewhat facetiously, "I've never lost a customer. Of course, if their methods didn't suit me I might 'fire' them." The article goes on to describe Kurt Froedtert as:

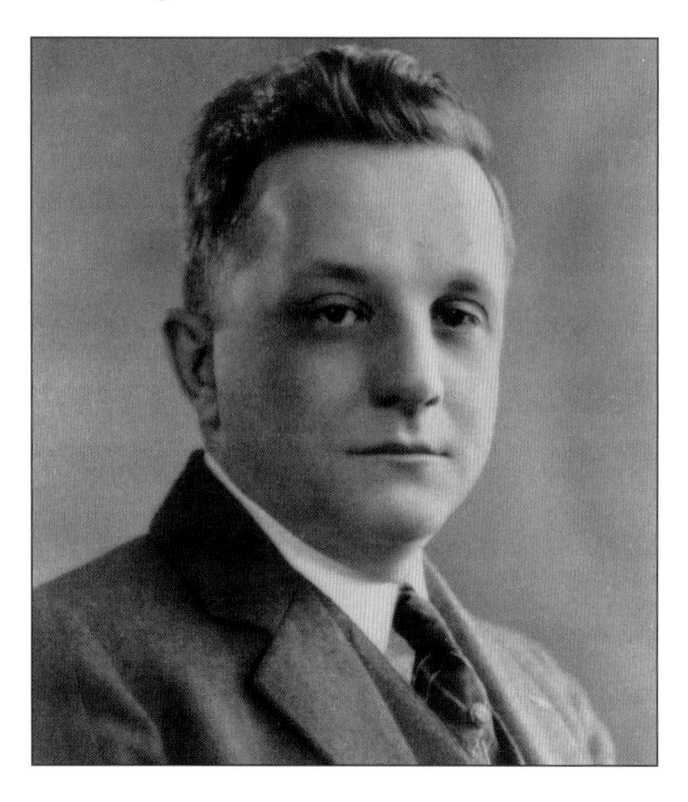

Kurt Froedtert at age 28

> ...a physically arresting specimen, sturdily built, powerful shoulders and arms and sensitive hands that never forgot how to play the piano, violin and guitar. Froedtert had a compelling personality that stood out in a group. He was a fluent talker, and expert teller of tales – none of them "blue" (risqué) – and for all his wealth, was not overbearing or the kind to push his weight around. He loved to discuss all manner of subjects and incited arguments to get other people's points of view, particularly on matters outside his own specialties.

That broad interest in outside matters set the stage for his business ventures into real estate, shopping centers, fisheries, oil, a cemetery, pharmaceuticals, and an abiding interest in conservation.

Froedtert's venture into the agricultural world is a prime example of his business sense. He bought seventy acres of land in Waukesha County on the Milwaukee County line, trying several ventures on the land with moderate success. When he realized that the Milwaukee metropolitan area was growing westward, where his land was located, he subdivided the property and sold lots at a handsome profit. His land holdings represented a substantial portion of the west sectors of Elm Grove. Today, Kurtis Drive and Froedtert Drive in Elm Grove are testament to his real estate acumen.

Kurt Froedtert was always moved to return his largesse for the community good. He loved giving gifts. Monfried's article relates stories of his penchant for gift giving:

> At Christmas he presented each of his employees, whom he knew personally, with a gift. In charities, Froedtert was generous but liked things done his way. He preferred to select his own beneficiaries. Froedtert was a member of Bay Shore Lutheran Church (Whitefish Bay). In one fundraising campaign

at the church he gave $20,000 – a sizeable gift at that time. When campaign donations slowed he offered to build several homes and permit the church to sell them and retain the profit. He was somewhat dismayed when the church leadership decided against entering the real estate business. It is said that Froedtert's attendance at Bay Shore Lutheran became less frequent, but he remained a devout man starting each workday with a prayer.

Over time, his own charitable foundation donated $150,000 for community improvements in Milwaukee, Detroit, Minneapolis, and Winona, Minnesota, cities where he had plants. In the year before his death in 1951, he gave $10,000 each to the Marquette University and University of Wisconsin medical schools for heart research. In the last year of his life, he donated another $10,000 to the Marquette University School of Medicine to support the teaching program in pediatrics. That interest and association in the field of medicine, backed by support for medical education, may have been a harbinger of what finally evolved from his last will and testament.

At the time of his death, the total value of Kurt Froedtert's estate was estimated between $9 million and $11 million. Fifty-four percent of that total was designated to establish the Froedtert Memorial Lutheran Hospital Trust. The remainder of his estate was left to his wife Mary, his two daughters Mazie and Suzanne, and a number of close friends and business associates.

The will called for a hospital to be named the Froedtert Memorial Lutheran Hospital. The wording in the will did indicate that the hospital should give preference to Lutherans but should be nonsectarian. In the years following Froedtert's death, national trends in the hospital industry, as well as tax and reimbursement rules, favored less restrictive policies in the makeup of administrations and boards of directors. While some board members at Froedtert Hospital may be Lutheran, there is no directive or mandate limiting membership to people of that persuasion. Historically board representation at Froedtert Hospital has been ecumenical. Since its opening in 1980, the hospital has served the needs of people of all faiths. ■

Chapter 2

Beginning the Long Journey

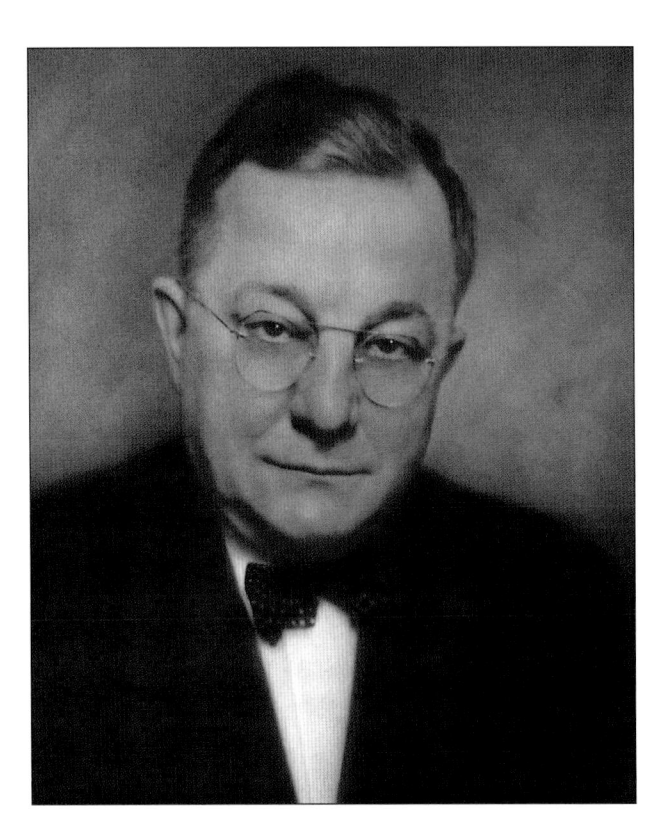

Kurtis Froedtert died of cancer on December 6, 1951. In the last year of his life, his gifts for medical research to the state's two medical schools were significant. His support for faculty development at the Marquette University School of Medicine established a relationship between the hospital trustees and medical education that eventually led to the concept and realization of an academic medical center. Those keystone gifts formed a bridge over which many would travel in the ensuing thirty years before the Kurtis R. Froedtert Memorial Lutheran Hospital would open in 1980.

The Froedtert Hospital Trust was a major gift to the community. In 1951, it was the largest individual bequest ever in Milwaukee's history. The story of Froedtert Hospital goes hand-in-hand with the development of the Milwaukee Regional Medical Center.

The hospital trust funds became available at a propitious time. Milwaukee and all of Southeastern Wisconsin had experienced major changes in medical and hospital care in the post-World War II years. This major trust fund represented a potentially significant catalyst for change in the organization and in the quality of healthcare resources for the region.

The Marquette University School of Medicine, long a beneficiary of Mr. Froedtert, was having financial difficulties in the early 1950s. An accreditation visit by the Liaison Committee on Medical Education in 1952 revealed two

Kurtis Froedtert

major deficiencies: the need for a stronger medical school faculty and money. The latter issue would lead Marquette officials to the Froedtert Trust in the hopes of obtaining financial support to increase the number of full-time faculty in both the basic science and clinical teaching programs.

In a paper later prepared for Marquette University and the Medical College of Wisconsin archives, Dr. John Hirschboeck, dean of the school, discussed the efforts of the medical school to raise the necessary funds:

> Father O'Donnell, Mr. Casey, Marquette's Vice President for Community Relations, and I were invited to spend a week as guests of the Froedtert Trustees in Bal Harbour, Fla., to discuss the possibility of collaboration between the Medical School and the Trustees in promoting medical education and research. . . . The Froedtert Trustees and Father O'Donnell and I concluded the meeting with an agreement that we would collaborate to create a medical center program and that we would enlist the support of others in working toward this end.

Attorney Joseph E. Rapkin was the personal counsel for Kurtis Froedtert from 1943 until Froedtert's death in 1951. A senior partner in the Milwaukee law firm now known as Foley & Lardner, Rapkin was one of four people named in the will as executors and trustees of the Kurtis R. Froedtert Memorial Lutheran Hospital Trust. The others were law partner Leon F. Foley; William Janssen, senior vice president of the Blatz Brewing Company; and Howard T. Ott, president of Wisconsin Memorial Park.

Probate work on the will was complex. Froedtert had invested in real estate and other ventures during his lifetime, and he was instrumental in building Southgate on Milwaukee's south side, the first shopping center in Wisconsin. Shortly before his death he had also begun planning for the Westgate and Northgate shopping centers. Westgate eventually became known as the Mayfair Mall, with Marshall Field's

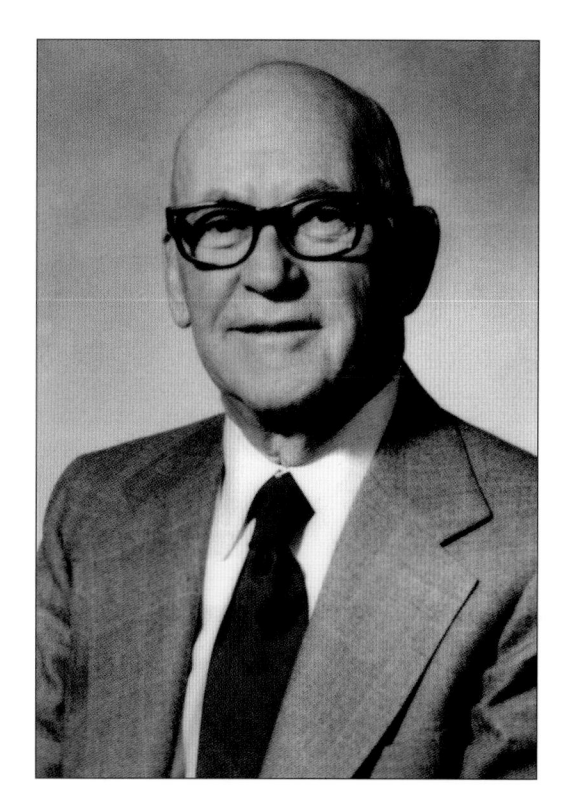

Attorney Joseph E. Rapkin

as an anchor store in the first move of that retailer outside the city of Chicago. Investments in Florida and local real estate, conservancy land, and the Wisconsin Memorial Park cemetery were among other assets of Mr. Froedtert's estate. At the time, these real estate investments limited the amount of funds available to plan and build the hospital.

The probate of Froedtert's estate would not be finalized until August 1956. While the will was in probate, the Froedtert Hospital trustees began to explore the best means to implement Froedtert's wishes. The trustees wanted to research the state of medical and hospital care in the community as it existed in 1951. They were especially interested in a study of the Marquette University School of Medicine and its impact on medical practice and hospital care in the community.

The inclusion of Marquette's medical school in this initial study held special significance. A medical school serves as a resource for medical manpower as well as the seat of research and new technology. The trustees knew of Froedtert's high regard for the school and its role in health education for Milwaukee.

The trustees also wanted to review the critical need for more physicians. At the time, the ratio of physicians to population served in Wisconsin was one of the lowest in the nation. The medical schools at the University of Wisconsin and Marquette University had limited capacities, turning out a combined two hundred graduates per year. Projected physician need would require both schools to double enrollments. Exploding technology in medicine required more scientists and full-time physician instructors to insure the highest quality medical school graduates. ■

Chapter 3

Surveying the Healthcare Landscape

To develop a medical center plan with Froedtert Hospital as a key facility, needs and opportunities had to be identified. Part of the planning process was to identify any difficulties. But no one could have predicted how substantial the difficulties would be in the years that followed.

The trustees first sought consulting expertise regarding patient care and the potential to support medical research and education. They hired Dr. Basil McLean, director of the Strong Memorial Hospital at the University of Rochester School of Medicine and Dentistry, to do the research. He was assisted by John T. Law. The study, which began in May 1952, evaluated the healthcare environment in Milwaukee with particular emphasis on the education and research components. The final report was issued nearly a year later in early 1953.

McLean noted the substantial number of solo physician practices compared to the larger physician group settings seen elsewhere in the country. He found the quality of care in the community hospitals to be

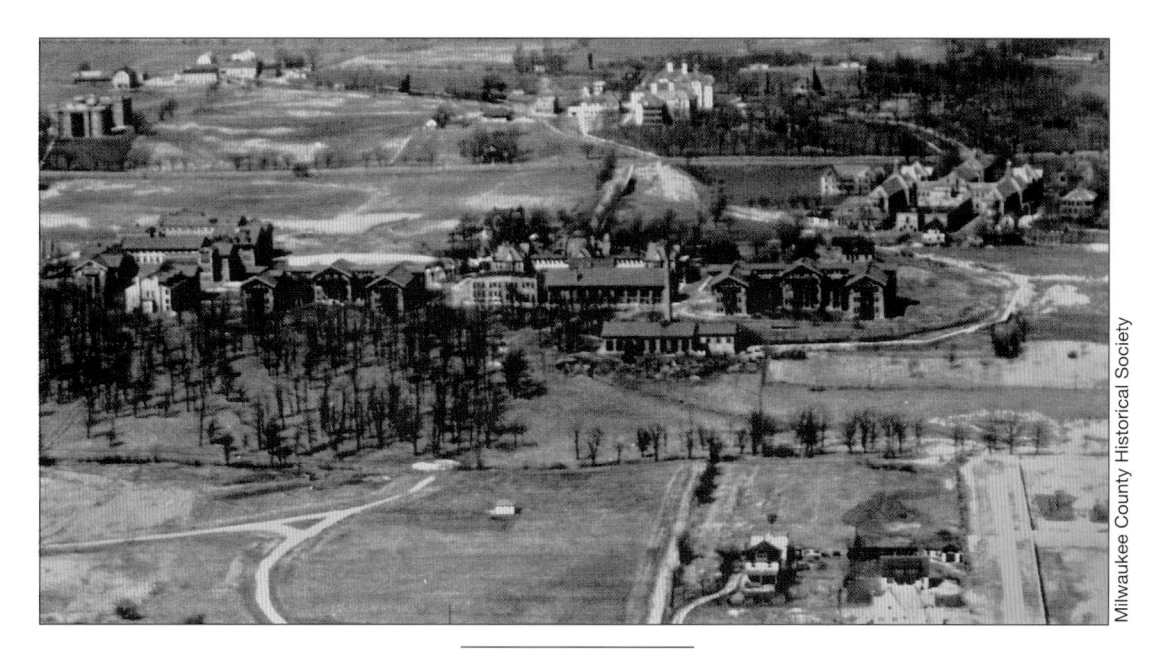

Milwaukee County Institutions Grounds

extremely capable. He noted that Milwaukee hospitals were relatively small and lacked outpatient facilities. But he was impressed by the Milwaukee County Institutions' facilities. His report noted, "The Milwaukee County Institutions have achieved a degree of development rarely found in the United States. They are impressive in size, beautifully landscaped, favorably located and are more comparable to university hospitals in many respects than any other general hospital in Milwaukee." This evaluation of Milwaukee County General Hospital and the other health services on the campus became a key consideration for the site of Froedtert Hospital and as a suitable location for a regional medical center.

At the time, Milwaukee County General Hospital had the area's largest post-

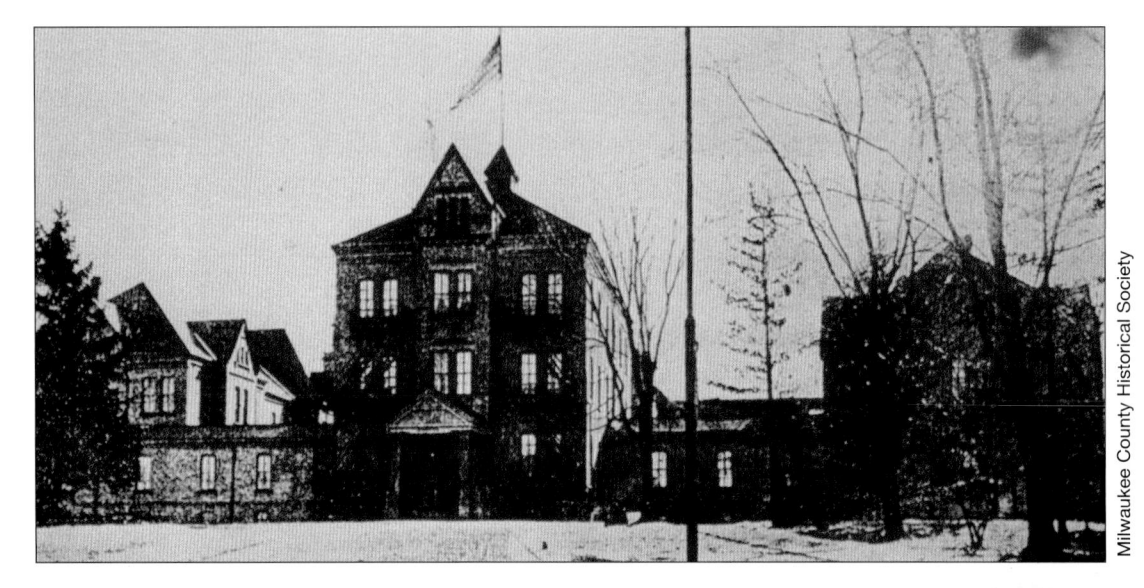

Original Milwaukee County Hospital

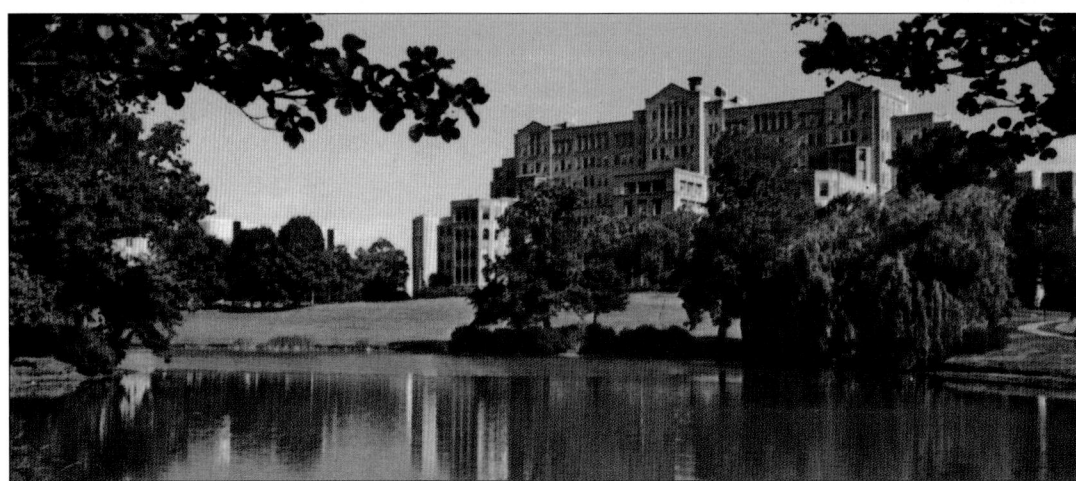

Milwaukee County General Hospital, 1927

graduate training program for physicians. The teaching program and house staff at County General that Dr. McLean found so remarkable played a major role in his recommendations for the best utilization of Froedtert's trust.

The strength of the County's teaching program can be traced to William Coffey, director of the County Institutions from 1915 until 1952. Coffey's administrative strength was his insistence on planning, coordination of services, and professionalism for all County health and social services. He convinced the Board of Administration for Health and Social Services to appoint Dr. Harry Sargeant as administrator of County General. Then Coffey and Sargeant persuaded Drs. Joseph M. King, a surgeon, and Francis D. Murphy, an internist, to serve as unpaid

William L. Coffey

As director of the County Institutions for thirty-seven years, William Coffey forged major reforms in the structure of Milwaukee's health and social welfare programs that remain in place to this day. His major changes in the organization, planning, and professionalization of social and health welfare services set the stage for the eventual creation of the medical center on the County Institutions Grounds. Mr. Coffey's concepts to expand and consolidate health and social services gained national recognition. Other local, state, and federal agencies adopted many of his program concepts.

A native of Milwaukee, Mr. Coffey was a graduate of Marquette University and earned a degree in Dentistry from the College of Physicians and Surgeons, the predecessor to the Marquette University School of Medicine. His dental career was shortened when he assumed responsibility for operating his father's trucking firm.

When the Milwaukee County Board of Administration was formed in 1915 to consolidate and administer the work of social welfare, Mr. Coffey was appointed as a community representative. He served as secretary to the Board of Administration and soon became the driving force in changing Milwaukee County's health and social welfare programs. Within six years he was appointed director of the County Institutions—a position he held until his retirement at age seventy-three in 1952.

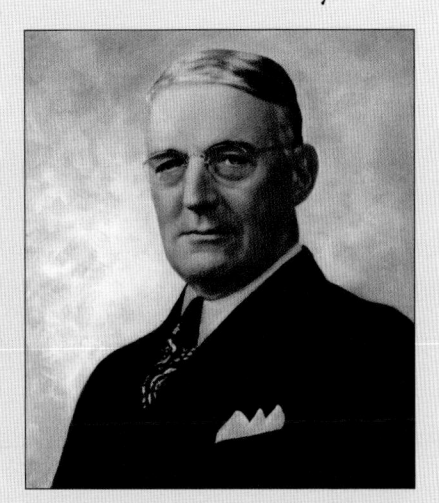

William L. Coffey

Mr. Coffey's initial efforts centered on attracting well-trained professionals to plan and manage social, physical, and mental health services for County residents. Most of these professionals donated their time and provided patient services unparalleled in the Milwaukee area. His interest and initiatives in medical education fostered broadened clinical experiences for Marquette medical students and expanded programs in postgraduate training for physicians in medical and surgical specialties. The County's School of Nursing was ranked among the best in the nation.

He served as Marquette's Athletic Board Chairman for thirty-eight years and was named the 1950 Alumnus of the Year in recognition of his extensive service to the school. Mr. Coffey was a widely recognized civic leader with a special interest in the American Red Cross. Each of his ten children received university degrees and went on to specialize in areas including social work, education, medicine, law, engineering, allied health sciences, and religious life.

volunteers to direct the surgical and medical services and programs at County General. This triumvirate of Drs. Sargeant, King, and Murphy was largely responsible for developing the hospital undergraduate and postgraduate surgical and medical teaching programs as early as 1928. Unfortunately, none of these men lived to see the fruits of their labor develop into a major academic medical center. The programs they established were the keystones for the highly successful teaching programs on this campus today.

In his report, McLean expressed concern about the financial difficulties Marquette's medical school was encountering and cited the national respect that the school had earned over the years. He emphasized the value of the university to the community in terms of its intellectual and cultural contributions. McLean said Milwaukee was fortunate to have Marquette University and its medical school, concluding, "The advance of medicine and medical practice in Milwaukee must be tied to and can exist only if the medical school is strengthened." Despite the school's financial difficulties, McLean's report praised Dr. Hirschboeck in his efforts to build a full-time basic science and clinical faculty.

Harry W. Sargeant, MD

The widely recognized and long-held reputation of excellence in patient care at Milwaukee County General Hospital rests on the shoulders of Dr. Harry Sargeant. This quiet, self-effacing man was the hospital's administrator for forty years.

A native of Long Prairie, Minnesota, Dr. Sargeant was a 1914 graduate of the College of Physicians and Surgeons in Milwaukee and completed his surgical residency at County Hospital. World War I interrupted his pursuit of a surgical career when he served overseas as a captain in the U.S. Army Medical Corps. After the war, he returned to County Hospital as a staff surgeon.

Dr. Sargeant became a key figure in the restructuring of health services when he was appointed administrator of Milwaukee County General Hospital in

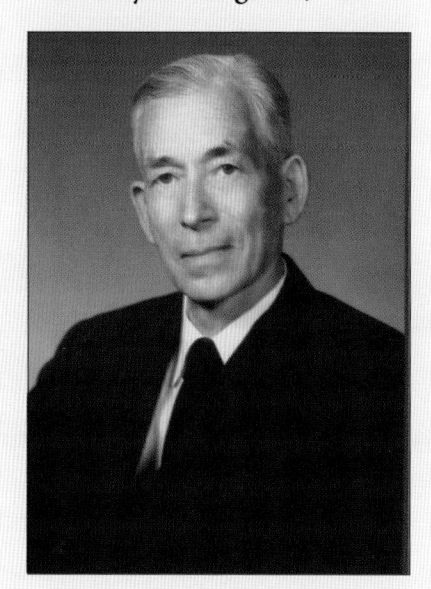

Harry W. Sargeant, MD

1922. His engaging personality enabled him to recruit community physicians as a volunteer medical staff for County Hospital. This highly qualified staff of physicians and surgeons served as the base for the growing medical education programs that Dr. Sargeant developed at County Hospital. Within the first decade of his administration, County Hospital's teaching programs for physicians, nurses, and allied health professionals became the largest in Milwaukee.

This sterling reputation for patient care and education at County Hospital impressed the medical center's planning consultants, who found County Hospital's education programs equal to those of many university teaching hospitals in the country. County Hospital's prized capabilities in patient care, education, and research became a principal element and focal point for the establishment of today's medical center on the County Institutions Grounds.

In his summary, McLean recommended:

> Froedtert Hospital be of moderate size containing approximately 100-150 beds; that its primary purposes be teaching and research. It is recommended that in the selection of professional staff of the Froedtert Memorial Lutheran Hospital, a close affiliation be maintained with the Marquette University School of Medicine and that the Froedtert Trust provide continuous financial support to the hospital.

These conclusions fit precisely the views and visions expressed a year earlier by Dr. Hirschboeck and the trustees in the meeting at Bal Harbour, Florida.

The McLean Report got a lot of publicity. Discussions were held among the Marquette medical faculty, Marquette University officials, Froedtert trustees, and the Greater Milwaukee Committee. An association of civic and business leaders interested in strengthening the quality of life for Milwaukee and the region, the Greater Milwaukee Committee played a quiet but effective role in the rescue of the

---

Francis D. Murphy, MD

Milwaukee County General Hospital's tradition of healthcare has been served by many individuals; notable among them is Dr. Francis D. Murphy. A native of New Diggings, Wisconsin, Dr. Murphy graduated from the Marquette University School of Medicine in 1921 and received his clinical training at Milwaukee County Hospital. His talent as a physician was recognized early in his career when he was appointed clinical director of medicine at Milwaukee County General Hospital in 1924 and chairman of the Department of Medicine at the Marquette University School of Medicine four years later.

A prolific writer, Dr. Murphy published numerous articles, including a series of Bedside Clinics based on cases he saw during rounds. He received wide acclaim for his clinical research on diseases of the kidney, including a 1933 Certificate of Honor from the American Medical Association for his work on Bright's Disease.

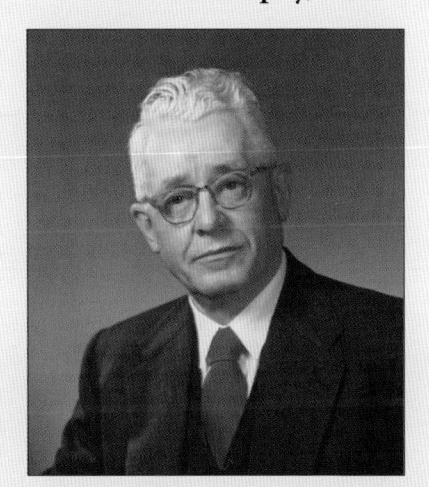

Beyond his individual accomplishments, Dr. Murphy's greatest contribution to Milwaukee County's healthcare tradition was his dedication to teaching.

Francis D. Murphy, MD

Throughout his career, he was committed to making ward rounds and fostering a dialogue among patients, students, and physicians. Students of Dr. Murphy's recall the way he inspired them to a level of emulation.

Dr. Murphy's desire to share his knowledge and experience was influenced in part by his love of books. Those closest to him recall the enjoyment and comfort he derived from the library in his home. It was, therefore, fitting that his contributions as a physician were recognized in 1959 with the designation of the Francis D. Murphy Medical Library at Milwaukee County General Hospital. At the dedication ceremony, many of Dr. Murphy's students and colleagues paid tribute to his years of service, including one student who testified that Dr. Murphy taught not only the science of medicine but the art as well.

Joseph M. King, MD

Dr. King spent the major share of his professional life at Milwaukee County General Hospital, where he served as a clinical professor and the director of surgery for thirty-four years. His interest and efforts in medical education were responsible for the growth of a postgraduate surgical training program at County Hospital that became the largest of its kind in the area. During his tenure at County Hospital, Dr. King trained more than 370 board-certified surgeons in the art and ethics of general and subspecialty surgery.

A graduate of the Marquette University School of Medicine, Dr. King began his residency in surgery at County Hospital in 1922. He remained there as a volunteer house surgeon until 1935, when he was appointed director of surgery and given part-time paid status. Dr. King did not view the responsibility to his patients and students as part time. Every night of the week, after a full day of surgery and teaching, he always made rounds visiting surgical patients at County Hospital.

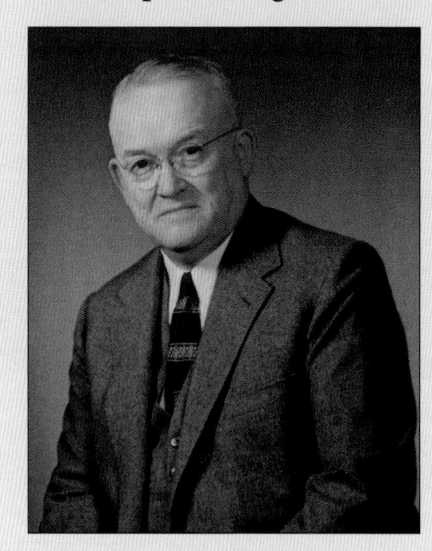

During his tenure, he envisioned the development of a major medical center and insisted upon including teaching facilities, classrooms, and research areas in the enlarged County Hospital facilities of 1957. He helped establish the Allen-Bradley Medical Science laboratory on the Milwaukee Regional Medical Center campus. Dr. King performed the first pneumonectomy—lung removal—in Wisconsin's medical history and developed a widely recognized technique for gastric resections. In recognition of his contributions in medical education, Dr. King received the Distinguished Service Award from the Medical College of Wisconsin in 1974.

An active alumnus of Marquette University, he was the team physician and a member of the school's Athletic Board for twenty-five years. He founded the Marquette University student health clinic and staffed that service for more than three decades. For his contributions and years of service to the university, Dr. King was named the Marquette Alumnus of the Year in 1967.

Joseph M. King, MD

---

medical school from its financial troubles. It would also wield influence on public and private resources to pursue the concept of a regional medical center.

A mutual sense of support had developed between the Froedtert trustees and Marquette's medical school. In February 1953, the Froedtert trustees and the Marquette University School of Medicine announced that they would create a teaching hospital and expand the faculty of the medical school. This was an informal, but fairly strong, relationship. On February 21, 1955, the Froedtert trustees and the Marquette University School of Medicine announced a plan to raise $300,000 annually for five years to expand and improve its faculty and to establish a teaching hospital in which the faculty would function as the medical staff of the Froedtert Memorial Lutheran Hospital—a key recommendation of the McLean Report. ■

Chapter 4

A Trust for the Future

In keeping with Kurtis Froedtert's original plan to ring the city with shopping centers, the attention of the Froedtert trustees in the mid-1950s was directed at construction of the westside shopping center. Income from this giant center in the path of westward growth for Milwaukee was viewed by the trustees as the source of capital to construct the new Froedtert Hospital. It was also viewed as a continuing income source for ongoing support for the hospital's patient service and teaching programs. Ground was broken for the Mayfair shopping center in 1956; it opened in 1958. However, it would take some time before Mayfair became successful as an income source that would generate the funds for construction of the hospital.

Even though the McLean Report of 1953 seemed to set the stage for where the future Froedtert Hospital would be located as a research and teaching facility, the trustees had an obligation to look at other options to carry out the terms of Froedtert's will. In this interim period, they considered an alternate site, the Milwaukee Sanitarium in Wauwatosa. Less than a mile from County General Hospital,

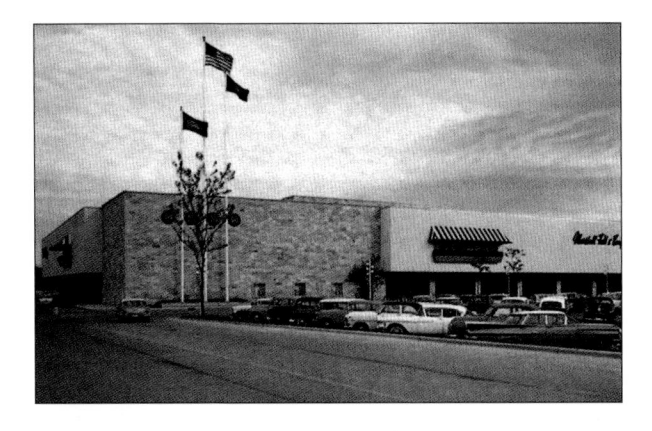

Mayfair Mall, 1959

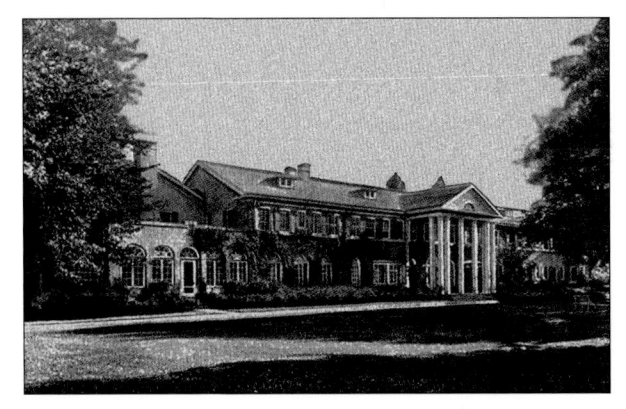

Milwaukee Sanitarium, Wauwatosa, Wisconsin

the Sanitarium had a 175-bed capacity with 300 full-time staff members, including eight full-time psychiatrists. It was felt that the proximity to the County Institutions Grounds would be workable within the medical center concept that Dr. McLean had recommended.

17

The Sanitarium enjoyed a national reputation as a for-profit private mental health facility. When the Milwaukee Sanitarium became a non-profit corporation in 1956, the board of directors was enlarged. New members included Dr. John Hirschboeck; Catherine Cleary, a First Wisconsin Trust officer; Mrs. Arthur Frank, a community leader; and Paul Pratt, president of Beloit College. These new members joined existing board members B.C. Bugbee, president of the Falk Corporation; Waldo Buss, executive director of the Sanitarium; attorneys Thomas Fairchild and Leon Foley; Dr. William Kradwell, vice president of Milwaukee Sanitarium; and Mrs. Gerhard H. Schroeder, president of the Sanitarium. Mr. and Mrs. Schroeder had operated the psychiatric hospital for many years.

The idea of locating Froedtert Hospital on the Sanitarium grounds occurred to Dr. Kradwell in 1955 when he read the trustees' plans for a teaching and research hospital. He discussed the matter with Mrs. Schroeder and Buss. They agreed. Subsequently the Sanitarium's Medical Advisory Committee concurred and recommended that it be pursued further.

By the fall 1955, Mrs. Schroeder mentioned the matter to the Froedtert trustees, who agreed to consider it. Dr. McLean was recalled to inspect the thirty-eight-acre Sanitarium site in Wauwatosa. The Froedtert trustees also visited the site and sought architectural review of its potential. All agreed that the proposal had merit.

With the approval of the Milwaukee Sanitarium's corporate members, directors, and officers, control of the psychiatric hospital was transferred to the Froedtert trustees in late 1955. This was done to facilitate the construction of Froedtert Hospital and the development of a broad medical program for Milwaukee. The new corporate title was Milwaukee Sanitarium Foundation, Inc.

As a long-time board member of the psychiatric hospital and one of the four Froedtert Hospital trustees, Leon Foley had hoped that the Froedtert Memorial Lutheran Hospital and the Milwaukee Sanitarium Foundation would become closely affiliated and eventually merge. With Dr. Hirschboeck's presence on the board of the hospital, a strong relationship developed between the psychiatric hospital and the Marquette University School of Medicine.

An announcement was made on Friday, December 16, 1955, that the site for the new Froedtert research and teaching hospital would be on the grounds of the Milwaukee Sanitarium Foundation, Inc., in Wauwatosa. Trustees then sought legal clarification to insure that each word and phrase of Froedtert's will would allow for construction of the hospital in Wauwatosa. A *Milwaukee Sentinel* news article of Saturday, December 17, 1955, indicated what the trustees wanted from the Milwaukee courts:

Sanitarium Site Urged For Froedtert Hospital

The Froedtert Memorial Lutheran Hospital, provided for in the will of the late Kurtis R. Froedtert, will be built on the grounds of the Milwaukee Sanitarium in Wauwatosa with the present sanitarium as its psychiatric division if County Judge Michael Sheridan rules that such a location meets the terms of the will.

An estimated five million dollars is available for hospital purposes.

Trustees of the hospital trust, set up in the will, revealed the choice of a location Friday when they asked for the ruling.

Atty. Joseph E. Rapkin, an executor of the estate and one of the hospital trustees, said the property was worth about a million dollars. He said the sanitarium officials had made the offer because they felt the institution could be operated more for the public good as part of the Froedtert hospital.

Judge Sheridan's interpretation of the will was asked because a clause in the will referring to the proposed Froedtert Hospital mentions that it was to be "in the city of Milwaukee"; the Milwaukee Sanitarium was in Wauwatosa.

By the following Monday, December 19, 1955, Judge Sheridan approved the selection of the Milwaukee Sanitarium as the site for the Froedtert Memorial Lutheran Hospital. The *Milwaukee Sentinel* coverage continued:

Judge Okays Hospital Site

County Judge Michael S. Sheridan Monday approved the selection of Milwaukee Sanitarium in Wauwatosa as the site for the Froedtert Memorial Lutheran Hospital. The judge swept aside any legal question as to whether the hospital could be built outside the city of Milwaukee.

"The general health, charitable and educational objectives and the intent of (the late Kurtis R. Froedtert) can best be served by the establishment and operation of the hospital at such time and place in Milwaukee county and in such manner as will stimulate progress in medical research and education as well as provide facilities for diagnosis and treatment," Judge Sheridan decreed.

The new affiliation and alignment of a teaching hospital on the Sanitarium site also met with the approval of community leaders and was reflected in a December 20 editorial in the *Milwaukee Journal* on the following day:

The arrangement by which the new five million dollar Froedtert Memorial Lutheran Hospital and the Milwaukee Sanitarium in Wauwatosa are to become one big medical project at the same location should be of great and increasing benefit.

The setup should be conducive to the closest teamwork in research, teaching and treatment by the medical staffs and the Marquette medical school faculty. That faculty will be operating the Froedtert hospital and already uses the County General hospital as a teaching center.

Again congratulations and thanks are due to those who are managing the Kurtis Froedtert estate, and to the Marquette University and medical authorities and others who have done so much to see that the Froedtert bequest brings the greatest good possible. They have earned honor for themselves, the university, the medical profession here – and for Milwaukee as a medical center of increasing importance.

Lending more weight to the new site selection was the creation of a Froedtert Hospital Planning Committee of Mrs. Schroeder, Foley, Buss, Dr. Kradwell, and Dr. Hirschboeck. This group held its first meeting in April 1956. That summer, Hirschboeck and Buss traveled to eighteen medical centers throughout the country, including Mayo, Yale-New Haven, Duke University, University of Michigan, University of North Carolina, and University of California-Los Angeles. But they did not see a prototype that would fit the needs of Milwaukee, its healthcare institutions, and the medical school.

Fundraising for the medical school and planning for Froedtert Hospital began to slow during 1957. Funds from the trust to construct Froedtert Hospital were not available because of the financial commitments to the real estate and shopping center projects planned by Froedtert before his death. While interest in the medical center concept—with Froedtert Hospital as an integral member—remained high, the pace slowed appreciably in the mid-1950s. Marquette University School of Medicine administration also faced financial constraints. Dr. Hirschboeck continued his efforts to build a strong basic science faculty and to add full-time clinical faculty members. The estimated budget for the faculty expansion was set at $300,000. ■

Chapter 5

In Pursuit of Funding

A federal program called Hill-Burton was enacted in 1947 to support construction and modernization of healthcare in postwar America. The program was administered through state government agencies. With the trust assets tied up in realty investments, the Hill-Burton program appeared to be a resource for funding to help build the Froedtert Hospital at the Milwaukee Sanitarium site.

Because a Froedtert Hospital corporation had not yet been formed, the Milwaukee Sanitarium Foundation, acting on Froedtert's behalf, submitted an application to the Wisconsin State Board of Health for financial support for the new hospital under the Hill-Burton program. The Wisconsin State Board of Health rejected the application in 1958, a definite setback for the hospital and the medical center plans. And more problems loomed. Some questioned the role of Froedtert Memorial Lutheran Hospital and its relationship to a medical school perceived as a Catholic institution. Other hospitals feared that the proposed medical center would compete for a limited number of patients in the area.

These concerns prompted the Froedtert trustees to form a committee of local physicians. Quite possibly, the trustees sought to cement better relationships with private practice physicians who would staff the hospital along with full-time medical school faculty physicians. They hoped that an integrated medical staff would engender community support for research and education in a regional medical center that would include other hospitals already involved in medical education.

Another interesting development surfaced. Some Milwaukee-area hospital representatives expressed a desire to affiliate or identify with the Froedtert Hospital Trust. St. Luke's and Lutheran hospitals, both with Lutheran ties, were among them. Both hospitals wanted to use funds from the trust for specialized services under the Froedtert name at their respective hospitals. However, the trustees rejected the idea. Years later, both hospitals would make separate and unsuccessful appeals to a newly formed Froedtert Hospital Board of Directors.

There was also the relationship to the Marquette University School of Medicine to be considered. Even though the medical school was incorporated separately from Marquette University, it was still viewed as a Catholic institution. For some, that affiliation was out of place.

To achieve the necessary cooperation among all parties in medical center development, the University Medical Center Corporation of Milwaukee was incorporated by Marquette University in 1958. It was to serve as an independent, non-profit body to bring about close institutional cooperation. Dr. Frederick W. Madison, a well-known Milwaukee internist long interested in a medical center, was appointed to this as a representative of the Froedtert Trust. He was viewed as the link between private practice physicians and full-time medical school faculty physicians who would staff the proposed hospital. Joining Dr. Madison on the new corporation's board of directors were Attorney Leon Foley, one of the four Froedtert Hospital trustees, and Dr. John Hirschboeck.

The University Medical Center Corporation of Milwaukee became a beneficiary under the will of retired schoolteacher Georgiana McFetridge, whose family owned a woolen company. The amount left to the University Medical Center Corporation was $25,000—a substantial gift in those days. The University Medical Center Corporation played a role in the development of the medical center plans, becoming the vehicle that community leadership used to keep the concept and value of a medical center alive. In the years ahead, it would evolve into the Medical Center Council, which administered medical center matters.

But opposition to the construction of Froedtert Memorial Lutheran Hospital was developing in local hospital and medical circles. The hospital and the medical center were now viewed as competition by other healthcare facilities in the area. To counter disagreement by the medical community and local hospitals, the Froedtert trustees formed another committee. Dr. Madison was named chairman.

The case for a medical center was again emphasized following a survey visit to the Marquette University School of Medicine by the Licensing Committee for Medical Education (LCME) in 1959. The LCME recommended that the medical school be fully and unconditionally accredited. However, the visitors expressed concern about the geographic distribution of facilities that were being planned in Milwaukee. As in previous reviews, the distance between the downtown locale of the medical school and its teaching affiliates with widely dispersed local hospitals was seen as a major drawback to a coordinated program of undergraduate and graduate medical education. ■

Part Two

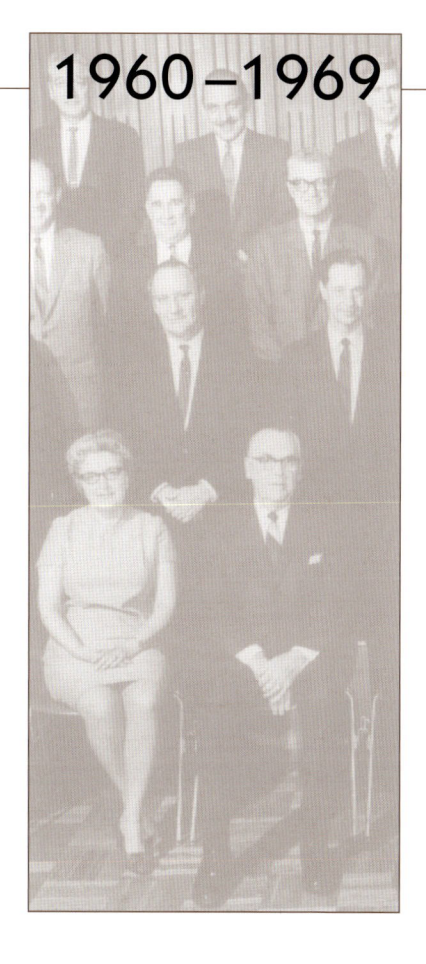

1960–1969

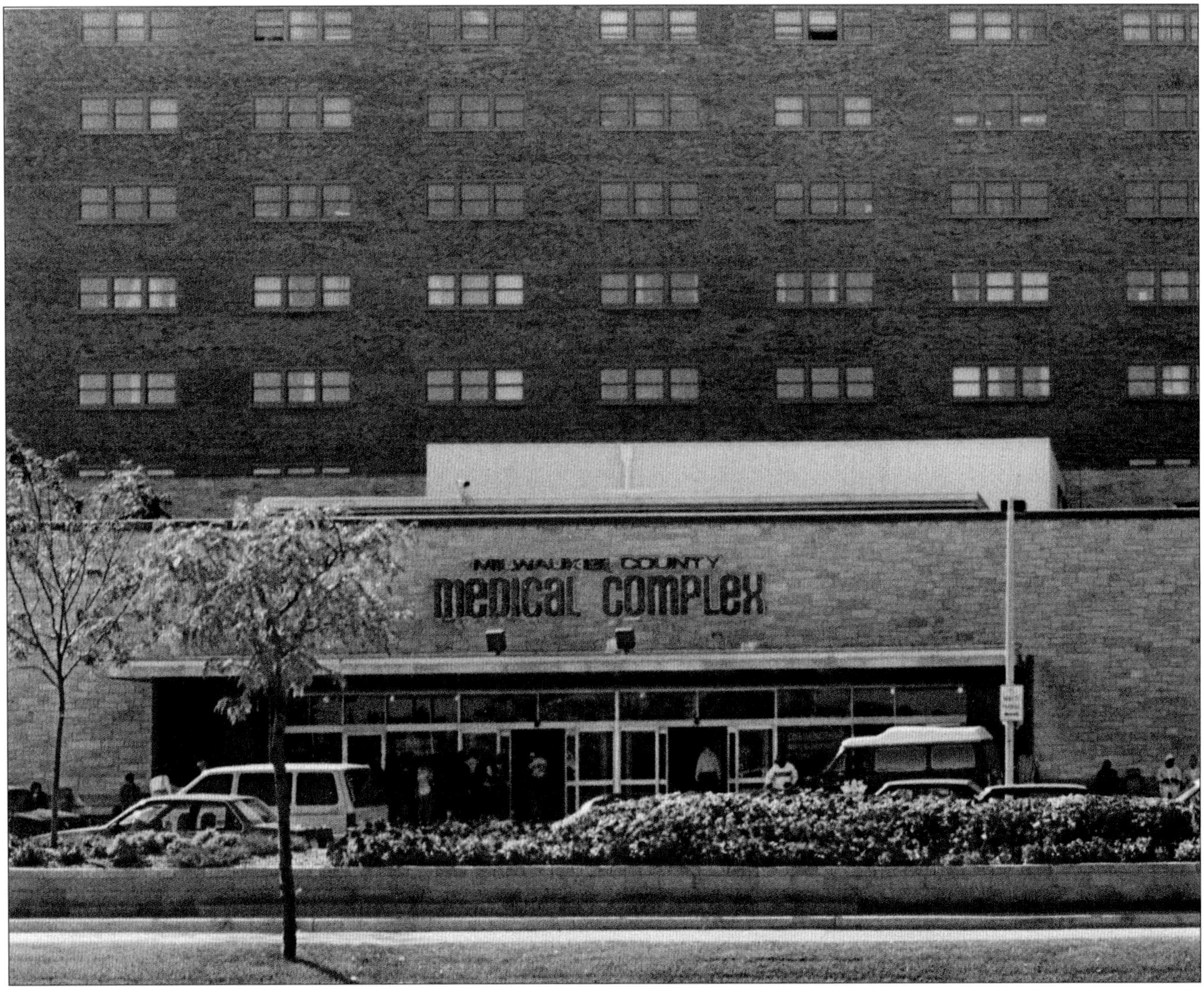
MILWAUKEE COUNTY
MEDICAL COMPLEX

Chapter 6

The Stage Is Set

From 1960 to 1970, Froedtert trustees faced a rapidly changing healthcare scene and political environment, beginning with a radical change in Milwaukee County government. John Doyne, longtime county supervisor and board chairman, was elected as the first county executive. Older County Board supervisors were replaced by younger individuals. Nationally, President Lyndon Johnson's "Great Society" plan brought about the Comprehensive Health Planning legislation of 1966. This legislation ushered in an era of regulations affecting health facilities nationwide.

These local and national developments caused some concern for the trustees who needed to know what effect these changes would have on Froedtert Hospital planning. McLean's study had recommended a teaching and research hospital as part of a medical center on the County Institutions Grounds. Another option was to locate the hospital on the Milwaukee Sanitarium campus.

It had been nearly a decade since McLean's study, and the healthcare landscape had undergone radical change. The trustees wanted an update on the local healthcare picture to insure that the hospital would meet community needs. In 1960, the trustees retained Dr. William R. Willard, dean of the Medical School at the University of Kentucky, to review medical education, research, and patient care in the region and to examine once again the County Institutions Grounds as a site.

Dr. Willard examined the relationship of the proposed Froedtert Memorial Lutheran Hospital and the Marquette University School of Medicine in terms of improved medical education, basic and clinical research, and advanced levels of patient care. He arrived at the same conclusions as Dr. McLean had in 1952. He did caution the trustees about possible community reaction to an arrangement between what was commonly perceived as a Catholic medical school in direct affiliation with a hospital bearing Lutheran in its title. The reaction to that affiliation was not too far off.

The trustees agreed with the Willard assessment that the Milwaukee County Institutions site was the most desirable one. The County Institutions provided

(opposite page) Milwaukee County Medical Complex, which was built in 1957

more land than the Milwaukee Sanitarium location. Then, too, sound teaching programs had been established at Milwaukee County General Hospital. The hospital could provide the necessary volume of patients, representing opportunities for clinical teaching in all medical and surgical disciplines, including mental health. Two potential sites were now available for Froedtert Hospital.

However, differing interests complicated the continued relationships among the Marquette University School of Medicine, the Froedtert Hospital trustees, and Milwaukee County government. There were no formal agreements. The medical school wanted to secure and finance a full-time faculty. County government sought to have a continuing and contributing presence in healthcare for the community—especially the indigent sick. Following the recommendation of the McLean and Willard reports, the Froedtert trustees wanted to establish a teaching and research hospital as part of a medical center. Added to these interests was the recommendation to centralize the medical school's basic science and clinical faculty in close proximity to the center.

Then another development emerged that had the potential to bring a vision to reality. . . . ∎

Chapter 7

Another Medical Center Site

While planning for the medical center seemed to languish, one more opportunity arose when the Veterans Administration announced that it would build a new hospital in Milwaukee to replace existing outmoded facilities. A tie-in with the Veterans Hospital loomed as a distinct possibility in 1960. The Veterans Hospital had been affiliated with the Marquette University School of Medicine since 1946, as part of a nationwide effort by the Veterans Administration to improve the quality of care. This affiliation with medical schools and other hospitals frequently included construction of Veterans Hospital facilities to serve as the nucleus of a university medical center at a single site.

Aware of this national trend, Drs. Edwin Ellison, medical school chairman of surgery, and William Engstrom, chairman of medicine, urged that the new Veterans Hospital be constructed on the grounds of the Milwaukee County Institutions along with the Froedtert Hospital and the School of Medicine Basic Science building.

Veterans Hospital was located at Wood, Wisconsin, a designated federal protectorate in suburban West Milwaukee. This site, which was in Congressman Clement J. Zablocki's district, had been in existence since shortly after the Civil War. Congressman Zablocki had campaigned for a new Veterans Hospital in his district.

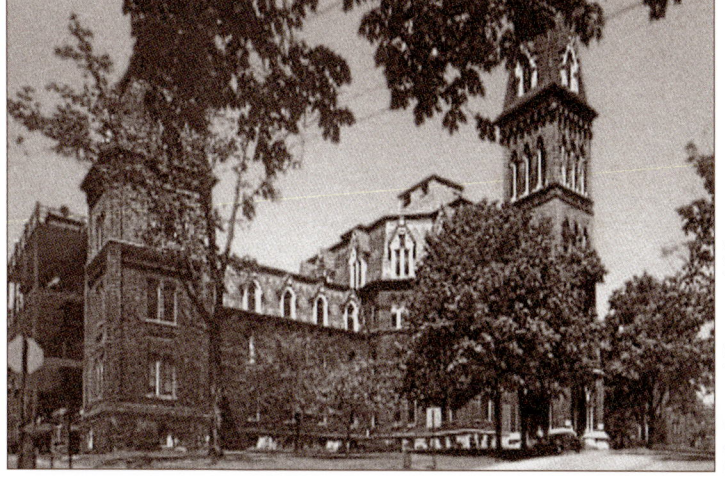

Veterans Hospital built in 1869, Wood, Wisconsin

At a public hearing held in the Milwaukee County Courthouse in early May 1961, Congressman Zablocki rallied veterans, including the American Legion and Veterans of Foreign Wars. It was standing room only. Also present were representatives of Milwaukee County government, the Medical Society of Milwaukee, and officials of Marquette University and its medical school. Dr. Hirschboeck presented the case for establishing the Veterans Hospital on the County Institutions Grounds. It would be alongside Froedtert Hospital, a new medical school, and the existing Milwaukee County General Hospital. Hirschboeck stressed that these facilities would constitute a major medical center that metropolitan Milwaukee needed. He further emphasized that a Veterans Hospital affiliation within an integrated academic medical center would benefit veterans by providing the highest quality of care.

The strength of the veterans' groups was evident. Congressman Zablocki stated the case for constructing the hospital at Wood, and vocal support for the new hospital remaining at Wood was loud and clear. At the courthouse that day, the proposal to locate the Veterans Hospital on the County Grounds died a sudden, but not unexpected, death. Eventually the Veterans Hospital was constructed on the Wood site, where it continues to function as a teaching affiliate of the Medical College of Wisconsin.

County Executive John Doyne was facing yet another problem: providing emergency services at County General Hospital. He felt that the tax-exempt status enjoyed by private hospitals should mandate their providing services to emergency cases. He said if private hospitals accepted emergencies, it would save county taxpayers $250,000 and that the County General Hospital could be closed. His comment appeared in the *Milwaukee Sentinel* on February 16, 1961. It may well have been the first public mention of closing County General Hospital. Doyne's perspective would change radically within a few years, and he would become one of the key factors in establishing a medical center on the County Grounds.

By the end of that year, Froedtert trustees made a formal and interesting presentation to the Milwaukee County Board of Public Welfare. They asked the board to consider placement of Froedtert Hospital adjacent to County Hospital and to retain the Milwaukee Sanitarium as a psychiatric hospital.

At that same time, Dr. Hirschboeck was dealing with growing turmoil between the medical school psychiatrists and the Milwaukee Sanitarium Board of Directors. By April 1962, the Milwaukee Sanitarium Foundation retained the firm James A. Hamilton and Associates to address the issues. The Hamilton consultant assigned to facilitate this six-month project was Dean K. Roe, who was positioned as the new chief executive for the Milwaukee Sanitarium. He was quickly approached by the Froedtert trustees to assist them with planning as well, so he assumed a joint role, and his engagement as the chief executive officer at the psychiatric hospital was extended.

On another front, the publication *Milwaukee Lutheran* began a series of articles questioning some of the past actions of the Froedtert trustees. In January 1963, the Lutheran Men in America of Wisconsin petitioned the courts to order compliance with the terms of Kurtis Froedtert's will. This began a three-year period of litigation between the trustees and the Lutheran Men in America over the plan to staff the hospital with faculty physicians from a medical school affiliated with a Catholic university. Four years later, this would no longer be an issue. Due to financial constraints, Marquette University would terminate its sponsorship of the medical school and the name of the school would be changed to Marquette School of Medicine.

The court action had some very positive aspects to it, however. As a result of the litigation, a formal organization was established for the hospital. ■

Chapter 8

Froedtert Hospital Corporation Formed

The Froedtert trustees and the representatives of the Lutheran Men in America reached a settlement in May 1965 to form a hospital corporation with a fifteen-member board, and the Lutheran men's organization and the trustees drew up a roster of prospective board members. The Kurtis R. Froedtert Memorial Lutheran Hospital Corporation was established on June 26, 1965. The new board would be responsible for the planning, organization, and fiscal integrity of the new hospital. but the assets of the trust would continue to be owned and managed independently by the trustees. The four trustees would have a voice but no vote on hospital board deliberations and decisions. This cooperative relationship and rapport between the trustees and the hospital board has continued since 1965.

The founding board of the hospital included seven directors from the Lutheran Men in America along with community representation. In 1965, Richard E. Vogt was elected the first president of the hospital board; William Jahn was chosen vice-president. Other members of the board included: Clarence Bickel, Harold F. Falk, Chester Foster, Arvid Frederickson, Arthur L. Grede, J. Martin Klotsche, William A. Seidemann, Reginald L. Siebert, Julien R. Steelman, Karl O. Werwath, John H. Paige, Ralph Ells, and Elmer Behrens. All held prominent roles in Milwaukee's business and industry circles.

Vogt's election as the first president of the board brought a leader with the

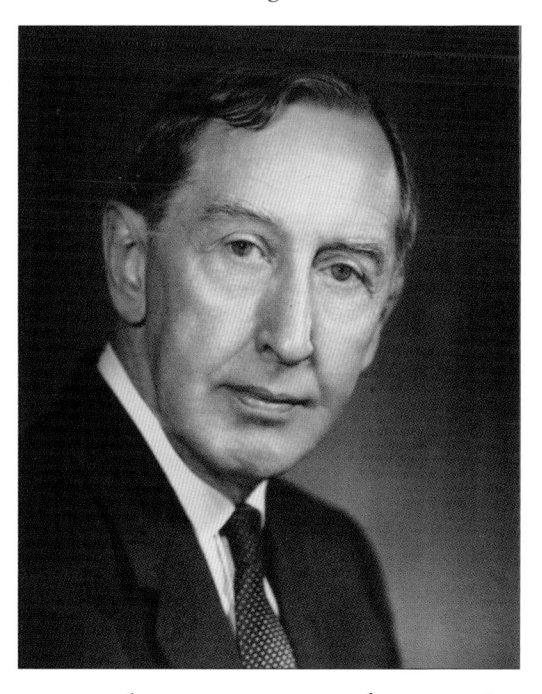

Richard E. Vogt, first president of the hospital board

30

patience, persistence, and perspective for determining just how and where Froedtert Hospital would fit into a changing healthcare scene. It was said that he spent more time on Froedtert issues than he did with his own business. The initial and subsequent diversity created balanced oversight and support of the hospital administration's planning and operating policies.

The formation in 1965 of the Froedtert Hospital Corporation and new board of directors could be likened to the arrival of a long-awaited relative. Board members were latecomers to a scenario that had begun as early as 1951. The newly formed hospital corporation now joined a "family" that had informally worked toward the creation of a medical center with Froedtert Hospital cast in a major role. The "family" that the new board members would join included the trustees, Marquette University School of Medicine, Greater Milwaukee Committee, Hospital Area Planning Committee, and Milwaukee County government.

Vogt had the vision and the character to establish a high level of leadership. His presence in the formative days of the hospital board could be called *providential*. This soft-spoken, self-effacing gentleman had the organizational skills, personality, and patience to forge deep and lasting relationships with Milwaukee's political and business leaders and healthcare administrators, earning their trust and respect. He set the stage by approaching each aspect of his and the board's responsibility with an open mind and a willingness to seek others' opinions. He viewed his and the board's responsibilities as legal and moral obligations to fulfill the terms of Kurtis Froedtert's will, independent of any outside pressures.

Aware of the need to have a fully informed board, Vogt orchestrated the early agenda of organization and planning. He set agendas so extensive that three organizational meetings were scheduled between August 5 and September 8, 1965. He worked tirelessly to communicate with each board member and sent daily mailings of information to his fellow directors. His personal goal was for the entire board to reach an optimal level of knowledge in the shortest period of time.

The chairman asked the new board members to list items for discussion. Major points included the organization, purpose, and operation of the new corporation; review of the settlement agreement with the Lutheran Men in America; and reviews of the McLean and Willard studies and of the Froedtert trustees' report to the Milwaukee County Board of Public Welfare. Board members were also interested in defining the characteristics of religious versus nondenominational hospitals and if a teaching hospital could be a good general hospital.

Among major concerns of the board was the Medicare/Medicaid legislation passed in 1966 that directly affected teaching hospitals. Prior to Medicare legislation, the only source of care for Milwaukee's indigent sick was Milwaukee County General Hospital. Under the Medicare/Medicaid law, patients could now choose to receive care at a private hospital. There was concern that a great portion of County's patients would choose to go elsewhere. Because that institution was identified as a key source in the establishment of an academic medical center, the loss of this critical volume of patients at County could also affect the proposed Froedtert Hospital's census.

The new board also considered the state law prohibiting the admission of private-pay patients to County Hospital, because County Hospital would not have the capability of serving private-pay patients to offset any potential loss of patients under Medicare. Without private-pay patients at County, the prospect of Froedtert Hospital getting referrals of patients with complex medical or surgical problems was in question. The advent of Medicare and the closer working relationship with the medical school made it apparent that for the difficult cases to be referred to a major teaching hospital, state law would have to be changed to admit private-paying patients to County Hospital.

Legislative change would have two positive results. Faculty physicians at County Hospital could bill for their services to private-pay patients, and this new source of income to medical school physicians would reduce the amount of tax dollars needed to maintain medical school physicians staffing County Hospital. Equally imperative was a change in state law to allow County government to lease land to private agencies. Changing the law was vital to the lifeline of the school and the hospitals and the related health services at the proposed medical center.

Once the organization of the new corporation had been completed, Vogt led an assessment of the local health scene. Local hospitals were contacted to see if the Froedtert gift could be utilized in concert with existing hospitals.

Two hospitals were particularly interested in the new hospital and in the decisions of the board. Lutheran Hospital of Milwaukee was one. Owned by the American Lutheran Church, it envisioned a Lutheran Medical Center on the Lutheran Hospital site. The plan called for additions that would give Lutheran Hospital a one-thousand-bed capacity. Froedtert Hospital would be a separate, but affiliated, specialty hospital within this Lutheran Medical Center. The other hospital, St. Luke's, suggested using the funds for its existing programs.

Vogt maintained close ties with Edmund Fitzgerald of the Greater Milwaukee Committee; Symond Gottlieb, executive director of the Hospital Area Planning Committee; and County Executive Doyne.

These contacts provided information on hospital and healthcare planning in Milwaukee. Within fifteen months, the new hospital board was ready to set its own compass heading to fulfill Kurtis Froedtert's vision. Vogt's legacy was the establishment of a standard of leadership that has continued over the years through each board chair's tenure.

The new Froedtert Hospital Corporation represented a potential teaching hospital for the medical school in the proposed medical center. However, the vision for the proposed center had become cloudy. Funding for construction of medical center facilities was questionable. The archival report of Dr. Hirschboeck stated, "The prospect for the development of the medical center, as originally conceived, began to decline and the Medical School began to look toward other possibilities including building its own hospital." In 1961, the medical school retained the services of James A. Hamilton and Associates, the hospital consulting firm that had been retained by the Froedtert trustees and the Milwaukee Sanitarium.

The Hamilton group's assignment was to cover all aspects of the master programming, planning, organizational, and physical development of the hospital. The idea behind retention of the Hamilton firm was to have sufficient data on hand as to what would be needed if the hospital were to become a teaching affiliate of the medical school. Douglas Kincaid was the Hamilton firm's consultant on this project. Working with him was Dean Roe, who continued to split his time as CEO at the Milwaukee Sanitarium and as a consultant for the new Froedtert Hospital Board of Directors.

Chapter 9

The Greater Milwaukee Committee and the Politicians

The Greater Milwaukee Committee (GMC) played a quiet, powerful, and consistent role in the development of the regional medical center and many other civic projects.

The GMC began before World War II, but its greatest impact occurred after the war. Some of its earliest projects included the Milwaukee Arena in 1950; the Milwaukee County Stadium, which brought the city's first major league baseball team in 1952; the lakefront War Memorial/Milwaukee Art Museum in 1954; and the new County Zoo in 1964. By 1969, GMC had been the impetus for nineteen major improvements in the community.

The GMC's secret to success was its ability to recruit a varied and talented group of key leaders in the city to carry out whatever projects the GMC felt to be in the community's interest and welfare. The medical center was one of many community endeavors undertaken by the GMC. The organization's usual strategy was to assign a GMC representative to a lead role to take a project to completion. Edmund Fitzgerald, retired president of Northwestern Mutual Life Insurance Company, led the medical center project. He is still recognized as one of the most influential community leaders in Milwaukee's history.

Substantial growth occurred in hospital remodeling, additions, and new technology after World War II. In this postwar expansion boom, hospitals sought charitable gifts from local business, industry, and private philanthropic foundations. There was little or no coordinated planning by hospitals in Milwaukee, and the demand for gift dollars was reaching a saturation point. Ultimately community leaders called for some type of organization that could assist hospitals in planning so as to reduce the duplication of health facilities and services and the constant appeals for money.

For the GMC, the solution to the planning and funding problems lay in the establishment of the Hospital Area Planning Committee (HAPC). This planning group was to oversee and coordinate the development of hospital facilities in Milwaukee. Within a few years the HAPC would become a fully funded planning agency under new federal health planning legislation.

In April 1965, University Medical Center Corporation President Dr. Hirschboeck arranged for a group of medical, business, civic, and hospital representatives to visit Texas Medical Center, which was considered the ultimate regional medical center operation.

Among the delegation that went to Texas were Dr. Gerald Kerrigan, the new dean of the Marquette University School of Medicine; County Board Chair O'Donnell; County Executive Doyne; Edward Logan, administrator of Children's Hospital; Dean Roe, CEO of the Milwaukee Sanitarium; and D.C. Firmin, administrator of the Veterans Hospital. Dan Patrinos, medical reporter for the *Milwaukee Sentinel*, accompanied the group. Following the trip, his newspaper articles did much to awaken and influence community leadership on the value of a medical center.

Edmund Fitzgerald

Today more people may recognize the name Edmund Fitzgerald as the huge ore ship that sank in Lake Superior more than thirty years ago. But Edmund Fitzgerald, the man, was a very big man himself. The president of Northwestern Mutual Life Insurance Company in the 1950s, he was born in Milwaukee in 1896. He served in World War I and graduated from Yale University. After graduation he went to work for Milwaukee Malleable Iron Company and was elected to the board of Northwestern Mutual in 1933. He became its chairman in 1958.

An active member of the Greater Milwaukee Committee (GMC), his "fingerprints are on almost every enduring civic investment," according to an article by Graeme Zielinski of the *Milwaukee Journal Sentinel*. "From the port of Milwaukee to the arts center, the post office to the War Memorial,

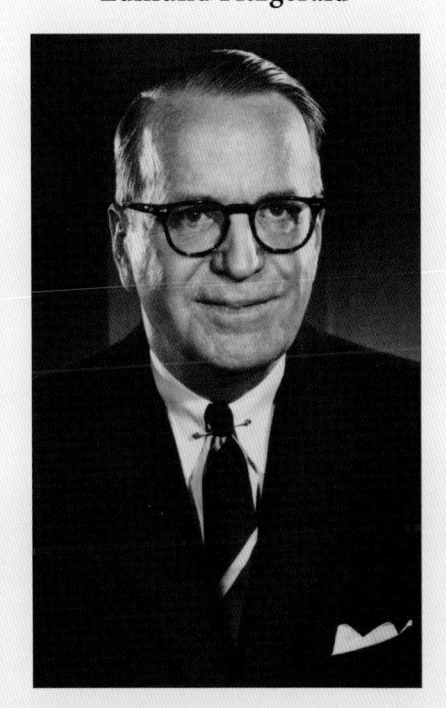

Edmund Fitzgerald

Fitzgerald was a 'one-man army'... for aggrandizing the city's institutions in the postwar period. He was a national innovator in healthcare provision, served on countless board and commissions, and was a strong patron of the city's arts organizations."

The Milwaukee Regional Medical Center was another one of many community endeavors undertaken by the GMC. The organization assigned Fitzgerald, the by-then retired president of Northwestern Mutual, to head the GMC's efforts to bring about the medical center. He also worked closely with Bud Selig to bring the Seattle Pilots to Milwaukee. The newly named Milwaukee Brewers brought major league baseball back to Wisconsin.

Fitzgerald, who died in 1986 at the age of 90, is still recognized as one of the most influential community leaders in Milwaukee's history.

His articles related the ability of a medical center to act as a magnet to attract the best medical practitioners, educators, and scientists to the city. Top-flight physicians would want to practice here. A center would also be a seat of research where discoveries or new technology and medical information could be put to use locally. Residents within the area of the medical center would have access to the best in medicine. The economic impact of the Texas center was that it created a boom in construction of offices, research centers, and hotel and motel business, as well as a means of providing job opportunities to local citizens. The involvement of community leaders was essential if the idea of a medical center was to move ahead. ■

Chapter 10

Enter the Political Leadership

County Executive John Doyne and County Board Chairman William O'Donnell played essential roles in maintaining the course toward the establishment of a major academic medical center. These two men of Irish descent had the political experience to push the center concept within County government.

Doyne, a native of Gary, Indiana, was elected as the first Milwaukee County executive in 1960. A graduate of the Marquette University Law School, he was a nephew of Willard "Mike" Lyons, longtime Milwaukee County supervisor and County Board of Public Welfare chairman. At the time, the County Board of Public Welfare governed the operations of the County Institutions with a fair amount of autonomy.

As a law student in the early 1930s, Doyne toured the County Institutions Grounds. He liked to recall that introduction to healthcare:

> I knew nothing of the County Institutions or the General Hospital, but my uncle took me out to the County Grounds and showed me all the facilities that were on

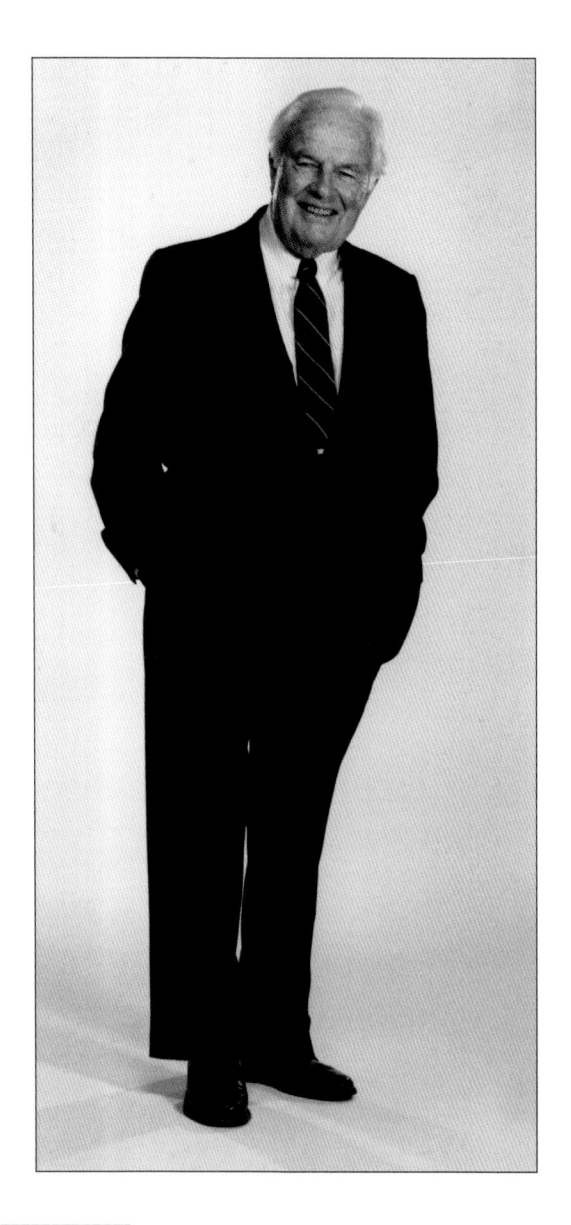

John Doyne, Milwaukee County's first county executive

that beautiful plot of land. As we walked around the grounds that day I remember him saying, "Someday this is going to be a great medical center." I never forgot that remark.

Doyne was a well-informed proponent of medical center organization. He liked to recall meeting Dr. Michael DeBakey, world-renowned heart surgeon, who was at Baylor University. DeBakey had been instrumental in convincing President Lyndon Johnson of the value of regional medical centers. During the Texas trip in 1965, Doyne met with DeBakey and told the surgeon of his desire to develop a major medical center similar to the one at Texas. Encouraged by DeBakey, he returned to Milwaukee with renewed interest in the medical center potential. He believed that existing community resources could establish a comprehensive, multi-institutional medical center to administer healthcare, education, and research in Southeastern Wisconsin. Doyne never lost sight of that goal.

In 1965, Doyne made his first move to involve both private and public interests in the eventual development of the medical center. In a meeting with Edmund Fitzgerald, he related his vision for a medical center. Fitzgerald, then the major power broker in the city, was equally interested in a regional medical center. Fitzgerald's interest in health and medical education stemmed from his association with Dr. Hirschboeck on the Community Welfare Council in 1948. After the meeting, Doyne invited local leaders to a community health and medical meeting.

The attendance at the October 6, 1965, meeting was a veritable who's who of Milwaukee leadership. Leaders from Froedtert, Veterans, Milwaukee Children's, and Milwaukee Psychiatric hospitals, along with Milwaukee County Institutions, were there. Milwaukee business leaders included Fitzgerald; Robert Foote, president of Universal Foods; Donald Abert, executive vice president of The Journal Company; Fred Lindner, vice president of the Milwaukee County Labor Council; and James Kelley, executive secretary of the Medical Society of Milwaukee County. Drs. Robert Purtell and James Sullivan, president and president-elect, respectively, of the County Medical Society, represented Milwaukee's medical community. Rounding out this panel were Hirschboeck; Kerrigan, dean of the Marquette University School of Medicine; Attorney Ted Wedemeyer; O'Donnell; O.W. Carpenter of Rex Chain Belt Company and chairman of the new Hospital Area Planning Agency; and Elizabeth Krzewinski, president of the Milwaukee Nurses Association.

Doyne told the group that an era of major and radical changes in the field of medicine and community health was underway at federal, state, and local levels. He cited the enactment of Medicare as one major change and stated that President

Lyndon Johnson earlier that day had signed the Regional Medical Program legislation. He added:

> The Milwaukee County area enters this interesting period with many plusses. There appears to be no serious shortage of hospital beds, when all of the present construction comes into use. We are justifiably proud of our public hospital. There is an established medical school and a superior group of physicians and surgeons. Our most serious concern, then, is related to the development of a medical center program and its relation to the already existing institutions, having in mind always to make available better care to more people.

The new Medicare and other healthcare legislation involved major changes in philosophy and responsibility. Doyne was aware of many controversial sources and that certain sections of the health services would react differently and advocate their special points of view. "The most important involvement in this problem must be the collective interest of the individual citizen and the public," Doyne stated. "It is my hope that a unified approach can be developed and lead to the formation of an active group dedicated to finding solutions within a reasonable time."

Doyne was empowered to appoint an executive committee to further plan for the regional medical center. He named Donald Slichter, president of the GMC; Fred Lindner, Milwaukee County Labor Council; Drs. Robert Purtell and James Sullivan, Milwaukee County Medical Society; Dr. Hirschboeck; Orville Guenther, director of County Institutions; O.W. Carpenter, Hospital Area Planning Committee; Dr. J. Martin Klotsche, chancellor, University of Wisconsin-Milwaukee; William Claypool, administrator, West Allis Memorial Hospital; and himself to the committee.

A steering committee included Edward Logan, Children's Hospital; D.C. Firmin, Veterans Hospital; Dean Roe, Milwaukee Sanitarium; and Drs. Purtell, Sullivan, Hirschboeck, Kerrigan, and Harold E. Cook, medical director of County Hospital.

In November 1965, Doyne's executive committee met with the Greater Milwaukee Committee and requested that the GMC assume a leadership role to develop a regional medical center for Milwaukee. The GMC accepted the assignment and established a Medical Center Study Committee chaired by Heil Corporation CEO Joseph Heil. It included Edmund Fitzgerald; John Nuzum, president of the First Wisconsin Trust Company; and Delbert C. Jacobus of the Jacobus Company.

The problem outlined by Doyne's steering committee was two-fold. The original McLean Report of 1951 noted that Milwaukee and Southeastern Wisconsin lacked a comprehensive medical center. Within that medical center void were the problems of the future of medical education, the growing complexity of medical care, and a forecast for a shortage of physicians and other healthcare professionals. The second leg of the problem was the rising costs of education programs for the health professions.

Under Heil, the study committee's approach was systematic and well planned. Before any detailed studies were undertaken, the committee outlined the essential characteristics of an academic medical center:

- A relationship with a first-rate medical school;
- High levels of specialization in all disciplines offering the broadest scope of services;
- A large, full-time medical staff relatively free from economic problems and drawn from as many medical and surgical specialties and subspecialties as possible;
- A large number of highly skilled scientists and specially trained personnel at the doctoral and predoctoral levels; and
- A scientific community to conduct research for the benefit of patients, physicians, and the community.

Chapter 11

Help from the Hospital Area Planning Committee

Although the Greater Milwaukee Committee had planning resources, it sought the expertise of healthcare planners. The details of this major study would be delegated to the GMC's Hospital Area Planning Committee (HAPC). Symond Gottlieb, executive director of the HAPC, had been a director of hospital and medical facilities and an administrator of Hill-Burton funding in Michigan.

The HAPC was the first group in Milwaukee to assess medical and healthcare needs, and its studies and recommendations affected the establishment of new services, technology, and facilities in the greater Milwaukee area. The committee had sizable "economic teeth" in its review process, such that project approval by HAPC staff and board usually won backing from Milwaukee's philanthropic resources. Hospital projects that were denied by the HAPC usually found that charitable contributions were hard to obtain, putting plans for expansion or renovation on hold. The HAPC assumed a formidable role in the GMC's medical center study and would continue to be a force in the 1960s and early 1970s on decisions about Milwaukee-area healthcare facilities and services.

As the federal government became more involved in healthcare planning, the HAPC evolved into a federally funded health systems agency, with significant power to review and judge the worth of any health programs or facility planning in the seven counties of Southeastern Wisconsin. The government's health planning agencies came to be viewed as either a blessing or a curse, depending on the approval or disapproval of a health facilities plan. In time, the Southeastern Wisconsin Health Systems Agency turned out to be a near-fatal element in Froedtert Hospital's fight to exist. As Froedtert wound through a maze of regulatory bodies on the local, area, state, and federal levels, there were other unforeseen obstacles.

The GMC Study Committee asked the Hospital Area Planning group to carry out a detailed study on healthcare, education, and research in a medical center setting. Milwaukee's health and business resources also became involved in the study. This coalition proved to be a textbook example of private and public sectors working together. In January 1967, the GMC presented the results of its study to County Executive Doyne. The major recommendations of the report stated that a medical center should be:

- a resource for the care of complex medical problems;
- a model of excellence in which physicians and other healthcare personnel can be adequately trained;
- available to all persons who require its services, regardless of ability to pay or place of residence;
- a focal point of scientific leadership that contributes to the excellence of the entire community's medical care program either directly or indirectly;
- able to demonstrate its capacity for broad service to the entire community;
- able to provide broad and intensive education programs; and
- a pioneer in the development and application of modern technology whose discoveries would be applied locally to enhance the quality of care throughout the community.

The Sunday, January 15, 1967, issue of the *Milwaukee Journal* carried the report as a front page story:

**Push Medical Center Now,
Milwaukee Leaders Urge**

Head of Committee Calls Project Vital to Well-Being of Citizens

The Greater Milwaukee Committee Saturday proposed immediate development here of a major medical center. Principal participants would be the Milwaukee County government, the Marquette University Medical School and its affiliated hospital and the University of Wisconsin.

The Medical Center would extend well beyond the metropolitan area. Its hub, however, would be the county institutions grounds in Wauwatosa, particularly County General Hospital.

Adjacent to the hospital would be built a new medical school basic science building, replacing the Cramer building at 561 N. 15th St. (on the Marquette campus) and a laboratory, research and private teaching hospital.

Under the plan, Marquette's medical school would be divorced from the university and affiliate with a medical center corporation. Autonomy for the school has already been proposed. A medical center corporation was organized several years ago.

The article quoted Carlton P. Wilson, president of the GMC. "We are convinced that the development of a major comprehensive medical center, including at least one first-rate medical school, is extremely important to the health and well-being of citizens in this area."

The McLean Report of 1953 and the Willard Report of 1960 were broad assessments of healthcare in Milwaukee. The GMC study, called the Heil Report, had greater detail and involved local healthcare people familiar with existing

The Heil Report

Marquette University created a separate School of Medicine on January 14, 1913. Dr. John Hirschboeck, dean of Marquette's medical school in the early 1950s, shared the commitment of the faculty and the community to maintain a strong medical school. But the financial difficulties that plagued the medical school in the 1950s and 1960s were a source of concern.

In 1952, Dr. Hirschboeck unveiled plans for an ambitious venture: the "University Medical Center of Milwaukee," the precursor of today's Milwaukee Regional Medical Center (MRMC). His vision of an academic medical center drew support from both the public and private sectors. Kurtis Froedtert was a major supporter, and ultimately his bequest for Froedtert Hospital helped the community realize that the dream of an academic medical center was within reach.

On September 30, 1967, Marquette University terminated its sponsorship of the medical school and a private, freestanding institution named the Marquette School of Medicine was established.

This was a key step in the realization of a "University Medical Center of Milwaukee." Milwaukee County Executive John Doyne and Edmund Fitzgerald, chairman of Northwestern Mutual Life Insurance Company and a member of the Greater Milwaukee Committee (GMC), shared Dr. Hirschboeck's commitment to the development of an academic medical center. In a public/private partnership, they appointed the Blue Ribbon Task Force, headed by Milwaukee industrialist Joseph Heil, Sr., to study the need and potential for an academic medical center in Milwaukee.

The resulting Heil Report was presented on January 14, 1967. This report called for major public and private financing and support for a comprehensive regional medical center with the medical school as its hub. Carlton P. Wilson, president of the GMC, explained, "We are convinced that the development of a major comprehensive medical center, including at least one first-rate medical school, is extremely important to the health and well-being of citizens in this area."

The Heil Report also prompted the medical school's board of directors to re-examine the independent institution's role and scope. The board determined that the medical school provided statewide services and, as such, should be named to reflect its ties to all residents of Wisconsin. On October 14, 1970, the board of directors voted to rename the medical school the Medical College of Wisconsin.

In the twenty-first century, the Milwaukee Regional Medical Center consists of six members: the BloodCenter of Wisconsin, Children's Hospital of Wisconsin, Curative Care Network, Froedtert Hospital, the Medical College of Wisconsin, and Milwaukee County Behavioral Health Division. The purpose of the MRMC is "to heal the sick, to teach the practice of medicine, and to advance medical science."

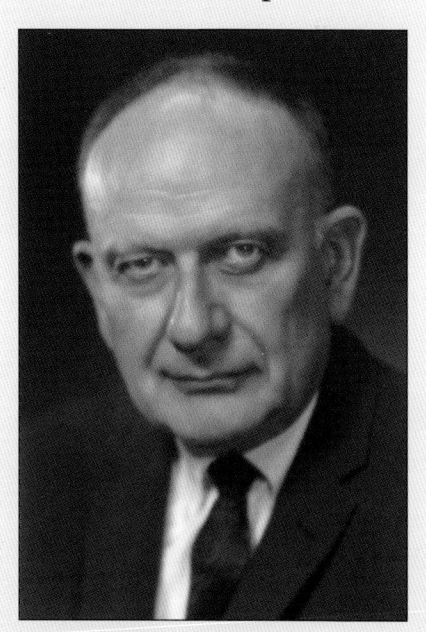

John Hirschboeck
Dean, Marquette University
School of Medicine

Medical Center Steering Committee

In 1968, the Medical Center Steering Committee consisted of a wide variety of representatives from business and industry, politics, medicine, and academia.

Top row: Leonard Alexander, DDS., dean, Marquette School of Dentistry; Symond Gottleib, executive director, Hospital Area Planning Committee; Gerald Kerrigan, MD, dean, Marquette Medical School; Martin Klotsche, chancellor, University of Wisconsin-Milwaukee; Edward Bachhuber, MD, associate dean, Marquette University School of Medicine; and Rudolph Schoenecker, executive secretary, Greater Milwaukee Committee.

Second row: Edward Logan, president, Milwaukee Children's Hospital; E.D. Klag, administrator, Veterans Hospital; I. A. Rader, Greater Milwaukee Committee; George Collentine, MD, Milwaukee County Medical Society; John Cowee, vice president, Marquette University; and James Sullivan, MD, Milwaukee County Medical Society.

Third row: Edmund Fitzgerald, Greater Milwaukee Committee; Frederick Lindner, vice president, Milwaukee County Labor Council; Charles Landis, MD, director, Milwaukee County Mental Health; John Petersen, medical director, Milwaukee County General Hospital; Robert Purtell, MD, president, Milwaukee County Medical Society; and Francis Rosenbaum, MD, Milwaukee County Medical Society.

Bottom row: Judge Ted Wedemeyer, Elizabeth Krzewinski, executive director, Visiting Nurse Association; Delbert Jacobus, Regional Medical Center Board member; Milwaukee County Executive John Doyne; Milwaukee County Board Chairman William O'Donnell; Joseph Heil, Greater Milwaukee Committee; and Edward Krumbiegel, MD, Milwaukee Health Commissioner.

community health resources that might be incorporated in a medical center. These local healthcare professionals helped identify research facilities and scientists and specialized healthcare programs. The structure, organization, and space for medical and health service education became a key issue as well.

The GMC Study Committee, with HAPC cooperation, concentrated on institutions that were affiliated with the Marquette University School of Medicine. These were: Milwaukee County, Veterans, and Children's hospitals; and the Milwaukee Sanitarium, by then known as Milwaukee Psychiatric Hospital; and the Blood Center. Other community institutions could seek incorporation into the medical center through major and minor affiliations and integrated programs.

Historically the Greater Milwaukee Committee was an action-oriented group. At the completion of the medical center study, the GMC sought to structure groups that would move on the medical center concept and get the job done. The GMC urged that planning begin as soon as possible to construct an adequate Basic Science building, sufficient laboratory research facilities, and a private teaching and research hospital on the County Institutions Grounds. The latter recommendation followed the findings of the earlier studies by McLean and Willard and insured a spot for the new Froedtert Hospital in a medical center plan.

One of the final recommendations sealed the private/public sector relationship. The HAPC and the GMC felt that implementation of the medical center program would have to include Milwaukee County and Marquette University officials. The GMC advised the County and Marquette to form a Milwaukee Medical Center Steering Committee to rapidly implement the recommendations of the report. It would be the overall governing body of the medical center, receive and disburse funds, and work out agreements with the institutions that would be part of the center.

Doyne appointed another group of thirty-three to the Milwaukee Medical Center Steering Committee, which Delbert Jacobus headed. He and a small group kept the planning effort on track. The group included Edmund Fitzgerald; Dr. Gerald Kerrigan, associate dean of the medical school; Dr. Harold E. Cook, Milwaukee County General Hospital; and Dr. John R. Petersen, director of Medical Services at County Hospital.

Doyne moved to determine the County Institutions' role as a key element of the proposed medical center as recommended by the Heil Report. Dr. Petersen recalled Doyne's reaction to the Heil Report:

> The development of regional medical centers nationwide and the Medicare and Medicaid legislation were seen as the basis for reexamining the County Hospital's role in healthcare in a way that would support developing a medical center. John Doyne felt that the federal programs of Medicare and Medicaid would relieve the County of much of the responsibility to provide all the care for the indigent.

With the expected relief, Doyne assumed that County Hospital could then broaden patient care, education, and research programs. Envisioning the hospital as the nucleus for medical center development, he requested that the hospital staff prepare a report as to the implications of the Heil recommendations.

The report emphasized the long history of Milwaukee County General Hospital as a major teaching facility for Marquette University medical students as well as its respected and long-standing programs in postgraduate medical education. This affiliation was viewed by staff as an established nucleus for a major medical center. The findings of the staff indicated a need to upgrade the County Hospital's facilities and services, which would require an outlay of more than $24 million—a hard sell to County supervisors. Of nine projects listed in the report, the highest priority was a 300-bed wing to replace more than 350 beds in the old 1927 hospital facility. The estimated cost of this wing was $9 million.

At the time of this report, the Froedtert Hospital Board of Directors had made no commitment to locate the hospital on the County Grounds. Some observers might have viewed the Froedtert Hospital Trust funds as a possible answer to the County Institutions' capital expenditure needs—especially the 300-bed wing. There is a view held that the eventual construction of Froedtert filled the need for the $9 million, 300-bed wing at the County Hospital. From another perspective, Froedtert Hospital's construction could be considered a $9 million savings to county taxpayers. ■

Chapter 12

Pursuit of Froedtert's Goal and Purpose

While the lifesaving efforts for the medical school were underway in 1967, the newly formed Froedtert Hospital Board of Directors continued to review a number of options for the best possible use of the hospital's trust funds. In June, the board scheduled a two-day symposium to consider earlier proposals by St. Luke's Hospital and Milwaukee Hospital (by then known as Lutheran Hospital). The symposium drew Froedtert board members and trustees, representatives of Marquette University and its medical school, consultants from James A. Hamilton and Associates, and two well-known national figures, Dr. Alton Ochsner of the Ochsner Clinic in New Orleans and Robert Fleming of the Mayo Clinic in Rochester, Minnesota.

Lutheran and St. Luke's hospitals both had Lutheran church sponsorship and were interested in some type of affiliation with the Froedtert Hospital Trust. Lutheran Hospital officials proposed that the funds be used to construct a women's hospital. The Lutheran medical staff and administration felt that a women's hospital on site would serve as a center for highly specialized care for complicated OB/GYN cases. This service represented an excellent teaching source. Teaching relationships with Marquette's medical school already existed. Lutheran Hospital's four-year surgical residency was the only one of its kind in the city.

The excellent teaching potential at Lutheran could have been a seed for a downtown medical center near the Marquette University School of Medicine on North 15th Street. Deaconess, Mount Sinai, Children's, and Misericordia hospitals were within walking distance.

St. Luke's Hospital proposed a "Partnership in Health." St. Luke's, which had more than five hundred beds and a broad service support system, suggested an automated health examination and multiphasic screening laboratory similar to a system at Mayo Clinic. This concept was rather limiting in that the Froedtert Trust money would be used for programs rather than a hospital facility.

The Lutheran Hospital proposal appeared the most workable because the concept included a separate building and identity. But because Kurtis Froedtert's will called for a general hospital, the Froedtert Board of Directors thought the Lutheran Hospital proposal was too restrictive. They also cited the recommendations from the 1953 McLean Report to give the new Froedtert Hospital a unique identity as a teaching and research facility within an academic medical center. The board vetoed both presentations and in 1968 retained a hospital architectural firm.

The Froedtert Board of Directors concentrated on the role of the hospital as a teaching affiliate of the medical school. Dean Roe completed a study in mid-summer of 1968 that sealed the interest of the Froedtert Board in an affiliation with the proposed medical center. On December 6, 1968, the Froedtert Board voted to name Dean Roe the hospital's administrator.

Roe's study concluded that Froedtert should be a private, independent nonsectarian hospital for the diagnosis and care of the sick. The hospital was not to confine its role to be one or several departments of another hospital. As an independent facility, its board would govern its financial affairs, administration, admissions policies, and appointments to its medical staff. The study recommended that patient care should be enhanced by a strong program of medical education and medical research in close affiliation with the medical school. Finally, it was recommended that Froedtert Hospital announce its intention to become a geographic or a community member of the medical center and to participate in the planning of the center. ■

Chapter 13

Medical School Faces Crisis

As plans for the medical center were developing, however, the financial plight of the Marquette University School of Medicine threatened its viability and continuance as the keystone of the proposed medical center. In the early 1950s, the Accreditation Committee of the Association of American Medical Colleges considered the school's financial resources inadequate and placed the school on "confidential probation." By 1960, the accumulated deficit for the school was $1.2 million. University and medical school officials felt that a new and major source of stable income was needed if the school was to survive as part of Marquette University

The problems of the medical school had come to a head. Father John Raynor, S.J., president of Marquette University, and Dean John Hirschboeck considered as one possible solution the sale of the school to the University of Wisconsin.

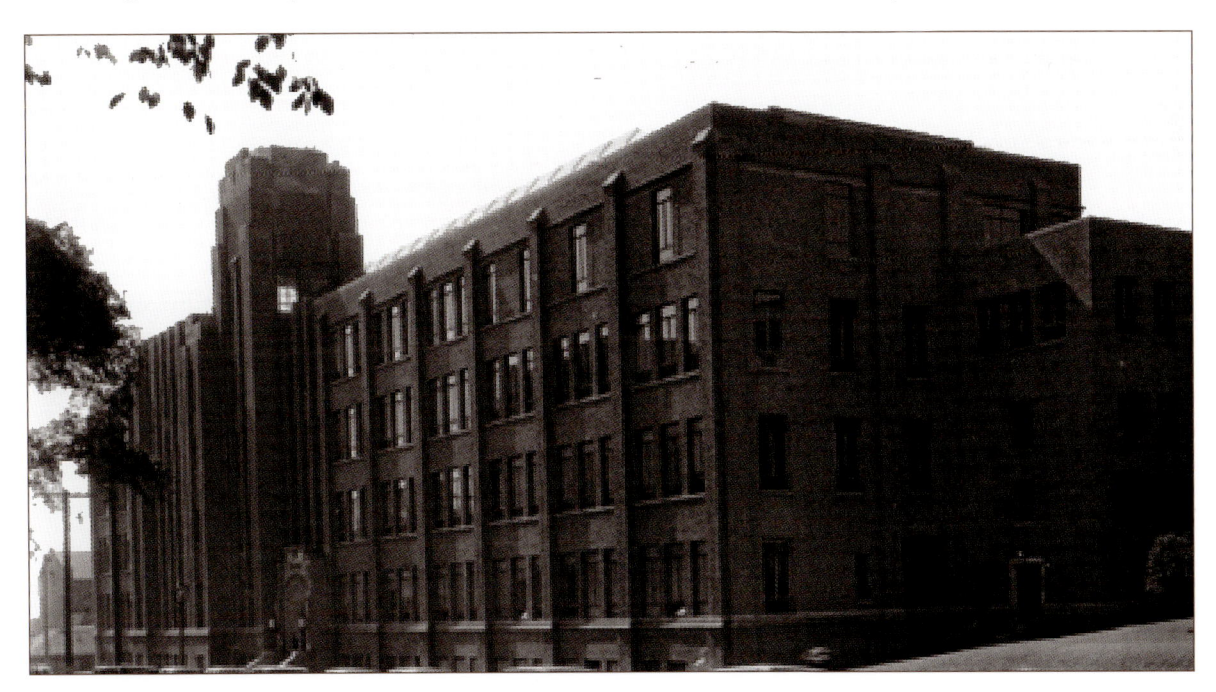

Marquette University School of Medicine

Another possibility was state funding for the school. The crisis turned out to be a blessing in disguise. The question posed —and legally untested—was whether state funding of any religiously affiliated institution was legal. To reduce complications, Marquette's legal counsel advised separation of the medical school from the university. The suggestion picked up considerable weight when the Lutheran Men in America threatened a suit to prevent tax money from being used for a school affiliated with a religious institution. On September 30, 1967, Marquette University terminated its sponsorship of the medical school. A corporate reorganization established the medical school as a private, freestanding institution named the Marquette School of Medicine.

At the same time, the State of Wisconsin was facing an alarmingly low ratio of physicians to population. Governor Warren Knowles established a statewide Task Force on Medical Education to study the needs. In late 1967, the Task Force recommended expansion of first-year medical school enrollment at both medical schools in the state to solve the physician shortage. It was clear that to handle the increased enrollments and keep its programs going, the now freestanding private Marquette School of Medicine would need state funds. By late 1968, the legislature's Joint Finance Committee declared that state support of the school would be in the public interest.

Despite this good news from Madison, the medical school still faced an immediate financial crisis. By mid-July 1968, Dean Kerrigan, who had succeeded Dean Hirschboeck in 1965, had sufficient money to continue operations for just thirty days. The school was in danger of closing for lack of funds.

The GMC again came to bat with big hitters. Robert Stevenson, who had been elected chair of the board of directors of the Marquette School of Medicine, and Joseph Heil, chair of the Medical Center Study Committee, acted as co-chairmen of a $600,000 fund drive sponsored by the GMC's Citizens Committee to save the medical school. At this point, it was the hoped that the favorable judgment of the State Supreme Court on the test case would clear the way for the legislature to okay state funding for the private school.

The fund drive was eminently successful. Full-page ads asked Wisconsin physicians to contribute. A flood of checks poured in from physicians throughout the state. Corporate foundations, major companies, and some wealthy individuals made significant contributions. The fund drive succeeded in raising more than $1 million.

At the end of October 1968, the governor signed an appropriations bill for the medical school for $1 million. The highly successful fund drive the previous summer, along with the state funding, saved the medical school and kept alive the idea of a regional medical center.

With the medical school financially sound, officials began planning a new $31 million Basic Science building adjacent to County Hospital. At the time, there was an expectation that the medical school would receive a $15 million grant under a federal program providing construction funds for medical schools and hospitals. A grant of this proportion would pay half the costs of the school's Basic Science building. These construction grants were a key element in federal legislation designed to establish regional medical centers nationwide. However, following on the heels of a second fund drive for the medical school came near-disastrous news— the $15 million grant from the federal government went elsewhere. The news from Washington cast a pall over what had been a euphoric atmosphere. The fund drive went to "time-out" status, and new problems began to develop.

At the same time, the makeup of the Milwaukee County Board of Supervisors had changed. Supervisors who favored the concept of a medical center had been replaced by new faces, and not all of the newcomers were as enthralled with County Hospital's role in a medical center. All the essentials of an academic medical center were detailed in a master plan developed by New York consultant Eugene Rosenfeld. Some of the newly elected supervisors viewed the master plan as a "pie-in-the-sky" concept.

In 1970, Democrat Patrick Lucey moved into the governor's seat after defeating Madison businessman David Carley. Carley's loss in the gubernatorial race was another blessing in disguise. In 1975, he became president of the Medical College of Wisconsin, the successor to the Marquette School of Medicine. Carley was the first chief executive of the school who did not possess a degree in medicine but held a PhD from the University of Wisconsin. ■

Part Three

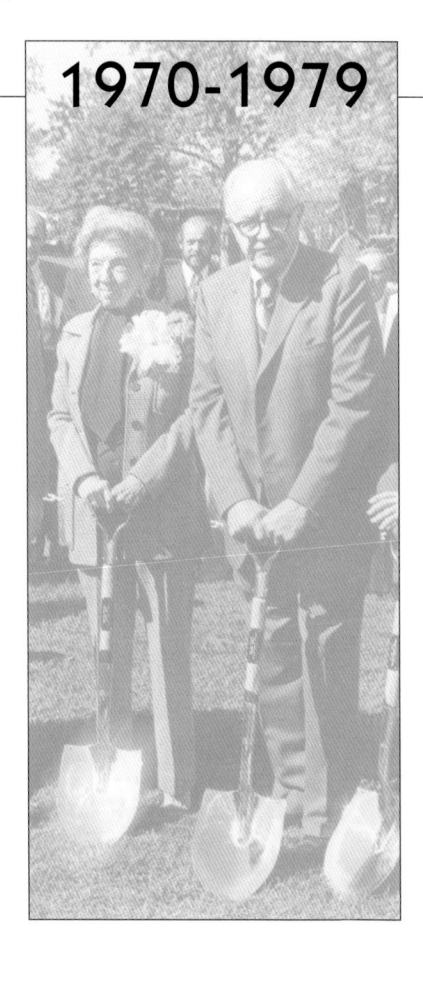

1970-1979

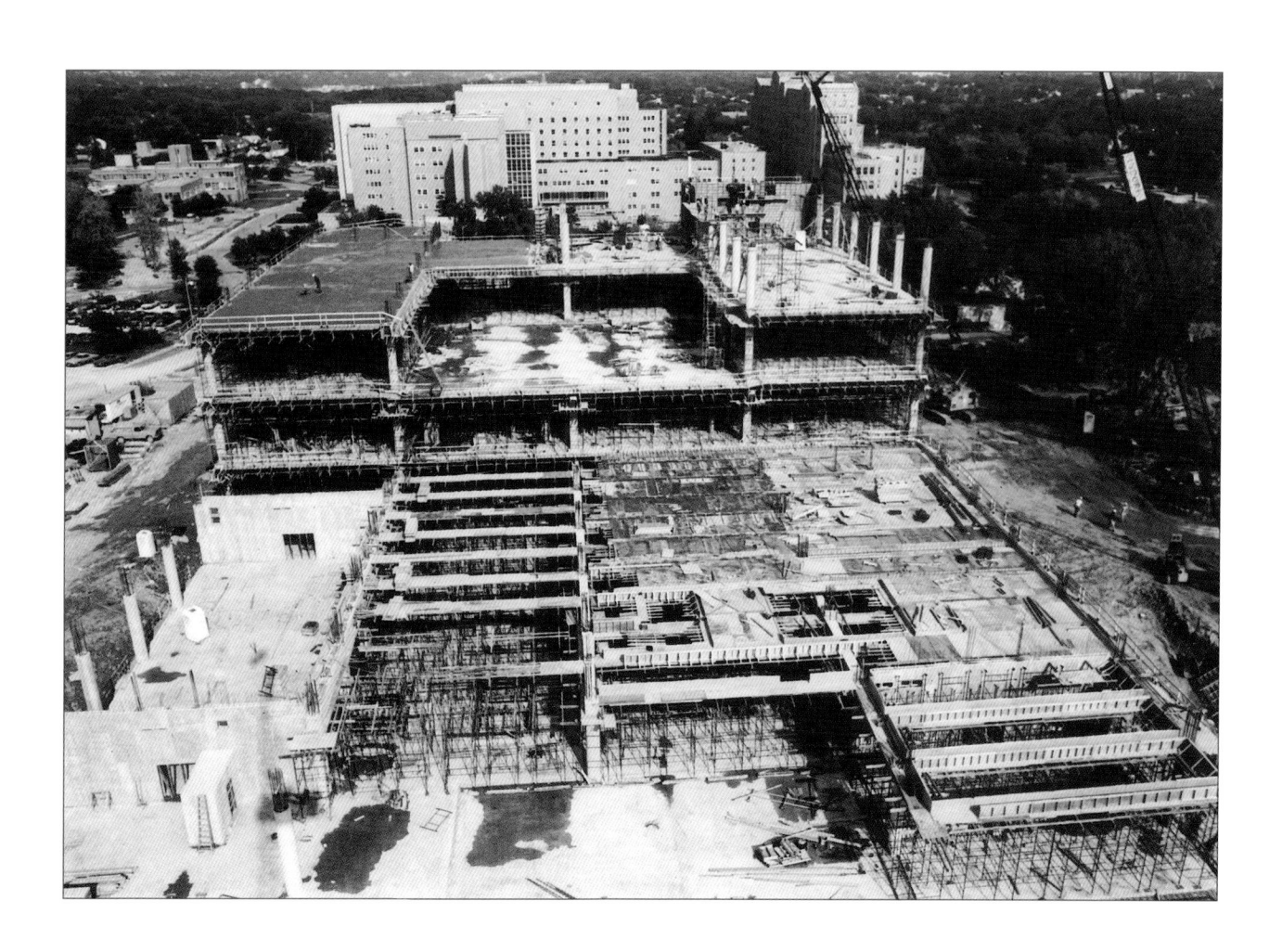

Chapter 14

Into the Turbulent Seventies

In Milwaukee's history, few endeavors generated as much turmoil as the development of the Milwaukee Regional Medical Center. The prolonged tussles between County officials and the private agencies, at times, seriously threatened the establishment of the medical center on the County Institutions Grounds. The 1960s and early 1970s were an era of major change in healthcare services nationwide, with new systems of health delivery being planned and designed. The fairly heavy hand of the federal government in healthcare planning had a direct bearing on the establishment of the medical center. Within this changing scene, unforeseen struggles developed locally as private and public agencies grappled for control of the planning and governing process of the proposed medical center.

Obtaining a land lease on the County Institutions Grounds was the first task facing Froedtert and other non-County-owned, private geographic members of the proposed center. It was a multi-step process. In any action involving health or social services with the County government, negotiations began with the County Board of Public Welfare. This quasi-public body of appointed community and County Board representatives was viewed as the "board of directors" for County facilities and programs. It had authority to establish budgets, policies, and administrative procedures for the County Institutions.

Welfare Board decisions were sent to the board of County supervisors. Ultimately a full board vote was needed for enactment after a review by one or more committees of the County Board, a system that is ponderous but essential in government. But board committees had the power to delay issues indefinitely simply by not scheduling a hearing.

State and federal approval of a proposed plan was another multi-step process. Applications for construction, renovation, new services, and technology often ran to more than one hundred pages. The professional staff of the area planning agency reviewed an application and then submitted it for further review by agency committees made up of healthcare providers and consumers. Public hearings and comments were required.

*(opposite page)
Froedtert Hospital under construction on the site of the County Grounds, 1978*

55

The plan was then submitted to the planning agency's full board for a vote. If approved, the application was submitted to the Division of Health Policy and Planning in Madison for final review. Any facility plan or program established without approval was subject to substantial fines and loss of Medicare and Medicaid reimbursement. The Comprehensive Health Planning Act of 1966 was legislation with teeth.

Despite the initial skepticism of some supervisors, in 1968 the County Board of Supervisors blessed the idea of the master plan. However, no formal resolution had been passed by this body—an oversight that would be a major point of contention a few years later. Support for the medical center from the new regime on the County Board was questionable, and the County Board of Public Welfare began to experience an erosion of its power to the more strident Health Committee of the County Board. The one constant in this 1970s evolution was the power and diplomacy of County Executive Doyne. He still held a strong hand, but it was challenged by the new faces on the County Board. ■

Chapter 15

The New County Board

Attorney Charles Mulcahy, a county supervisor from 1964 through 1976, described the local political climate of that time:

> The election of 1972 brought a new group of people to the County Board. The average age on the County Board prior to 1968 was 65-70 years. The old guard was gone and a new breed of members was elected. Several of them had previously served in the Wisconsin legislature, including Supervisors Sam Orlich, Michael Barron, and Richard Nowakowski. One of the life-long ambitions of Supervisor Nowakowski was to be elected chairman of the County Board. In the 1972 spring elections, Nowakowski became quite involved in the individual campaigns of prospective board supervisors and assisted many of them in their election efforts.
>
> Based upon the campaign activities of Mr. Nowakowski, those grateful supervisors elected him chairman on a 16-8 vote.

Mulcahy recalled:

> The eight supervisors who voted against his election as chairman were removed from positions of authority and responsibility. In their place Nowakowski appointed several supervisors he had actively assisted in their recent campaign efforts. A leading supporter of Nowakowski, Supervisor Terrance Pitts, was appointed chair of the Health Committee. This was highly unusual for a first-term supervisor. The Health Committee dealt with a wide range of complicated and complex healthcare issues. Supervisor Pitts immediately took political control of the situation. He was highly intelligent, energetic, talented, forceful, tough-minded, and demanding.

In retrospect, the role of the late Supervisor Pitts in medical center negotiations is understandable: it reflected his desire to insure that the citizens he represented had continued access to the care and employment opportunities that Milwaukee County General Hospital provided. In the end, as a member of the Health Committee, Supervisor Pitts cast one of the deciding votes to build Froedtert Hospital.

The Steering Committee proposed that the Medical Center Council should include representatives from each of the center's members. What lay ahead were more than a few battles between the Medical Center Council and County supervisors for power and control of the medical center's development. In the early 1970s, all of the players were already in place on the medical center stage. However, the script was only partially written.

The medical school survived its financial crisis and, as the Medical College of Wisconsin, was now a private, nonsectarian, freestanding institution. The Froedtert Board of Directors had reviewed numerous options and concluded that a teaching and research hospital within a medical center was the prudent move to make. The GMC experienced its usual successes: saving the medical school and pushing the medical center to a point of reality. Now the time had come to wrestle with the issues of providing healthcare in a fast-changing and regulatory environment.

On the local scene, Misericordia Hospital was in the process of building a new hospital in suburban Brookfield and closing its facility at North 22nd Street and West Juneau Avenue. Misericordia's move in 1969 to the west suburb with its new name, Elmbrook Hospital, reduced the total of central city beds. However, total acute care hospital beds continued to climb for the Milwaukee area. St. Joseph's, St. Luke's, and Columbia hospitals added more acute care inpatient beds. The so-called excess beds would play a major role in the approval process for Froedtert Hospital. Waiting in the wings on this stage was Dean Roe, who still held the chief executive post at Milwaukee Psychiatric Hospital. He would become a key figure in the negotiations for Froedtert Hospital's approval and in the organization of the Milwaukee Regional Medical Center. Roe would be in the midst of a confusing and complex plan to merge hospitals and pave the way for approval of the three hundred beds planned for the Froedtert research and teaching hospital at the medical center.

Major changes were taking place in government controls on healthcare planning and facility construction and services. Locally, the Hospital Area Planning Committee (HAPC) no longer could be considered a handmaiden of the Greater Milwaukee Committee, which had established and funded the local health planning agency in 1963. In 1971, it became a federally designated health planning agency known as the Comprehensive Health Planning Agency of Southeastern Wisconsin. Its jurisdiction included Milwaukee, Racine, Kenosha, Ozaukee, Washington, Waukesha, and Walworth counties.

The federal government's role in healthcare through the Comprehensive Health Planning Act and the regional medical center legislation served as a catalyst for Milwaukee County Executive

John Doyne. In January 1972, Doyne proposed an economic impact study of a regional medical center to demonstrate that a medical center would have a positive impact on the area. The study was to be funded by the University Medical Center Corporation with $15,000 of the $25,000 left to that organization by Georgiana McFetridge. The gift from the University Medical Center Corporation had a condition attached—selection of the consulting firm to undertake the study would be made by John Doyne.

That brought reaction from the new County Board Chairman Richard Nowakowski. He was quoted in the January 19, 1972, *Milwaukee Journal* as saying, "I love John Doyne, as we all do. He's a dear sweet man who we all admire, love and adore. But letting Doyne determine who does the study is like putting the fox in charge of the henhouse." It was a challenge to Doyne's power, and Doyne prevailed as usual. The County Board voted for his selection of a consultant on a 17-7 vote. But the challenge for power by the board would not end at this point.

The economic impact study, completed by May 1972, indicated that construction of the proposed medical center would create two thousand full-time jobs. In addition, thousands of dollars in new tax revenue for Milwaukee County and Wauwatosa would be generated from increased property values, and the center was projected to generate millions of dollars in new retail sales each year in the metropolitan area. While employment and payroll would increase, the report indicated that the number of beds for patients would be reduced by 34 percent. Total inpatient beds in Milwaukee at this time numbered 3,195. Under the medical center proposal, area hospital beds would be reduced to 2,121 by cutting the number at County General Hospital and the North Division mental health facility. Bed reduction would become a key issue in the days ahead as planning for the center gained momentum.

As expected, Doyne was pleased with those findings. He hoped that the report would clear the way for approval of the medical center concept, which had been delayed by questions about its costs and impact. He was overly optimistic.

The report said that construction costs for the center would total nearly $112 million, of which $70.8 million would be privately financed and $41 million publicly financed. The $41 million figure was to be used for capital improvements for Milwaukee County facilities. The report stated that if the center were not built, modernization and expansion of existing facilities on the County Institutions Grounds would cost the County $36 million. The economic report on the medical center represented an increase of $5 million in public money. It was not clear in the report where the public financing would come from.

County officials had never before faced a public/private relationship of this magnitude. Entering a partnership with private facilities was a new experience that may have engendered an undercurrent of distrust between the elected officials and the private agencies. Current and future events were to prove that the relationships between the private and public sectors would not always be harmonious. Doyne's role was clearly cast as a negotiator in the mission to establish the medical center. ■

Chapter 16

Lining Up the Leases

Leasing public lands to private enterprises was without precedent in Milwaukee County history. As the landlords of public land, County officials rightfully felt a deep sense of responsibility to protect the public trust in this exceptional piece of real estate. In one sense, they probably felt a loss of control over this land through the leases to the private agencies. As a starting point, leases were drafted for the Medical College of Wisconsin and the Curative Workshop, an outpatient service center for patients with disabilities. For the most part, these were standard land leases that County officials thought would serve as a master lease for all of the participants in the regional medical center. That would not be the case, however.

On June 1, 1972, the County Board of Public Welfare unanimously approved leases with the Medical College of Wisconsin and Curative Workshop to build their facilities on the County Institutions Grounds. The leases were for fifty years at $1 per year with options to extend another fifty years. At this point, the Welfare Board's action had to receive County Board approval. And the route to the County Board chambers was through the Health Committee. The power struggle began. Negotiations would consume hours, days, and months before the private and governmental agencies reached agreement.

Under the leases approved by the County Board of Welfare, the Medical College Basic Science building had to be completed by June 1, 1976. Curative's completion date was set for July 1975, and construction had to begin before December 31, 1973. Part of the problem in coming up with acceptable leases was the question of who would be responsible for providing the utilities needed by the two institutions as well as other costs that would accrue as the center developed.

The approval marked the kickoff of the long-discussed Medical Center of Southeastern Wisconsin. But the Welfare Board's approval was only the first step. It was assumed that full County Board approval would come without a hitch. That assumption was wrong.

As new chairman of the Health Committee, Supervisor Terrance Pitts sought to have a more forceful role in health matters. He felt that all negotiations with private affiliates for leases in the proposed medical center would have to go through him and his Health Committee. It took four years to negotiate the master lease.

One of the major issues was the cost-sharing formula. The formula would allocate various costs for the utilities, roads, construction, and maintenance expenses necessary to provide and maintain the infrastructure of the medical center. Cost sharing turned out to be a major point of contention between the County government and the private sector members. Arguments would run on for months. It was one of many major problems and numerous delays that brought about an editorial admonition from the *Milwaukee Journal* on August 17, 1972:

Stalling on the Medical Center

Further County Board delay in approving leases for the proposed Medical Center on County Institutions grounds could jeopardize a $15 million grant to the Medical College of Wisconsin and several millions already granted to Curative Workshop. In the case of the college, the last chunk of federal money to be allocated for medical education in the form of direct grants will be sliced and distributed late this month or early next.

The college stands a good chance of getting its $15 million request if it has a land lease from the county for its basic science building. Without it, the college will have to line up for future money to be given as loans. Other time pressures harass the college. It is committed to the state to expand its freshman class from 111 to 167 and to vacate buildings it now occupies at Marquette University by September, 1975. Curative, occupying rented buildings on the west end of the Institutions grounds, is under pressure to use federal money already granted for building purposes, and could conceivably lose its funds without a lease.

To make a political football at this late date out of a project that stands to benefit the entire state by attracting and holding topnotch medical people, by expanding medical training facilities in the state and providing high level research programs, is tantamount to throwing the game. The concept of the medical center is the result of long and careful study going back to January of 1967. Economic feasibility and impact studies have shown positive implications. Support has come from prestigious hospitals and health organizations. The Milwaukee County Medical Society has advised all supervisors of its approval and support. The money is there. As for county expenditures, the estimated $40 million required to update and improve its own buildings over a 10 year period seems to be the same amount the county is now spending at the rate of $4 million a year, and even this need be spent only if the county wishes to maintain its hospital and programs at peak quality.

Approval of the 20 year master plan by the County Board is not essential to get the center moving. Parts of that plan could eventually be turned down without affecting the overall viability of the center. But the leases need to be approved to get the available money and begin. Stalling now is pointless and could prove expensive.

The negotiations with the Health Committee of the County Board became very heated at times. The problems were enumerated in an investigative news series written by *Milwaukee Journal* reporter Harry Pease. The five-part series ran from August 20–24, 1972. Pease's assessment of the medical center situation was well researched and covered all sides of the controversy. He outlined the definition of the medical center as a federation of private and public health institutions that agreed to coordinate programs while each retained administrative and financial independence. Pease wrote that one reason the development of the center was hung up could be attributed to the view of some supervisors that Milwaukee County was a majority partner, even though the private agencies would spend twice the amount already spent by the County on existing facilities on the County Grounds. The headline on the series guaranteed wide readership:

County Fiddles as Med Center Burns

The Milwaukee area can have more than $70 million worth of new facilities for healthcare, education and research on the County Institutions grounds in Wauwatosa within five years and without spending more than a pittance in local tax dollars. It can, that is, if a dilatory contentious and under informed County Board can bring itself to act September 7.

There is much more to the Medical Center of Southeastern Wisconsin than the buildings proposed for construction near County Hospital by non-governmental agencies, but the projects, in danger of being talked and studied to death at the moment, are to be located there.

The medical school had applied for $15 million in construction funds from the National Institutes of Health. Grants would be made in the fall. Without a lease, the prospect of obtaining these funds was in jeopardy. Curative had received $2.3 million in a local public fund campaign. Another $2.4 million in a federal grant was earmarked for Curative when a building site became available. So there was pressure on the medical school, Curative, and the elected County officials to sign the leases.

Private agencies voiced concerns about the clauses that the Health Committee was attempting to impose within the lease agreements. In the Pease newspaper series, Roe, president and CEO, stated:

> Neither the school nor Froedtert could live with the conditions they were trying to impose. The Medical Center is to be a working cooperative. That changes if the conditions of operation are controlled by the County Board through the lease mechanism. The existing agencies have won national reputations for excellence. No way are they going to sacrifice their autonomy.

At a meeting of the Health Committee Subcommittee held August 25, 1972, Chairman Pitts and several other supervisors insisted that the Medical College agree to a land lease that would limit the number of out-of-state students and assure that the school had an active minority recruitment program.

Within a few days, the Health Committee unanimously supported the Medical College and Curative leases. The Curative lease produced little discussion; compromises were achieved on the medical school lease. The restrictive features of the medical school's lease remained intact, however. They provided for penalties if the school failed to achieve freshman enrollments of at least 63 percent Wisconsin residents, or if it discriminated against prospective students based on race, creed, sex, political affiliation, or family.

Representatives of the independent and nonpublic medical center members were upset at the Health Committee demands. Privately some talked about the possibility of building elsewhere and leaving the County Institutions out of their plans. Then Supervisor William O'Donnell, a proponent of and the best-informed public servant about the proposed medical center, said, "Without the Medical College we're dead. I don't think we can, or should, operate an ordinary community hospital," O'Donnell was reported to say. "You would expect that more would be done for the people of this area—and I'm not just talking about the poor people, I mean all people."

Supervisor Pitts was considering a resolution to change the name from the Medical Center of Southeastern Wisconsin to the Milwaukee Regional Medical Center. The proposal made sense insofar as none of the surrounding counties of Southeastern Wisconsin had committed any financing to the center itself.

Pitts thought that the County should have a greater voice in the affairs of the geographic members. He felt that private facilities using the public lands should be prepared to pay a fair share. He did not say what he considered a fair share.

"They talk about $1 a year rent," Supervisor John J. Valenti is quoted in the *Milwaukee Journal* series by Harry Pease. "The medical school provides nearly all the doctors that staff County

Hospital at 50 to 60 percent of what we'd have to pay otherwise. Without them we'd be dead. I feel there is an urgent need for the center and I want to get all these roadblocks out of the way."

County supervisors expressed other concerns, including accusations of deception on the part of the County Institutions' administration, the medical school, and the Medical Center Council, and arguments over the placement of roadways, shared costs of utility construction, increased traffic, and the location of proposed medical center buildings recommended in the master plan developed in the 1960s and 1970s. Some supervisors thought the building placements would detract from the park-like surroundings of the two lagoons facing Wisconsin Avenue.

The outcome of the County Board vote was still in doubt. Another article in the *Milwaukee Journal* series looked at alternatives if the County said no to the leases. Again, the headline drew attention to the problem:

If County Says No, Medical Center Isn't Dead

If the Milwaukee County Board rejects the Medical Center of Southeastern Wisconsin or imposes conditions the private member agencies feel they cannot accept, the project will not necessarily die. Three other courses of action had been considered.

- Establish a campus for the Medical College of Wisconsin, the Froedtert Memorial Lutheran Hospital, Curative Workshop and the Milwaukee Blood Center at the Veterans Administration Center.
- Buy land for a campus and proceed without involvement of any government agency north of Marquette University.
- Abandon the idea of a campus entirely. Each participant that would acquire its own location and programs would be integrated even though the institutions were physically scattered.

Supervisor Charles Mulcahy became alarmed at the possibility of private medical center members moving to the VA or another site other than the County Institutions Grounds. "Supervisor Pitts wanted the County to control this process and allocation," Mulcahy recalled. "I felt that the private sector would never make the policy and financial commitments if controlled by the County." A long, difficult, and sometimes bitter series of negotiations and public meetings followed. The Health Committee was the forum for discussion between the parties.

County officials were angered by the turn of events that might lead to a mass exodus from the County Grounds to the VA site. Finally, after a heated, four-hour negotiating session with the County Board Health Subcommittee on August 25,

1972, the Medical College and Curative agreed on leases to build on the County Institutions Grounds. The full County Board would take up the Health Committee's recommendation for passage on September 7, 1972. Supervisor Pitts did not foresee any objections to adopting the leases as they had been hammered out in the committee meeting.

But new problems arose when the County Board's Health Committee recommended that the Medical Center of Southeastern Wisconsin be renamed the Milwaukee County Regional Medical Center. The Medical Center Council said that they saw no reason for a name change and felt that the County government was assuming a position as landlord to dominate a corporation in which the County itself was just one of eleven members.

Further, the formula for cost sharing for roadways, sewers, utility lines, parking, and clearing land for the proposed new facilities became a major point of contention. It was the core item that affected all of the geographic members of the medical center.

The Froedtert Hospital Board of Directors wisely defined the hospital's role and purpose as one of patient care, education, and research. At the Froedtert Board's request, Attorneys Maxwell Herriott and Robert Bradley, a Froedtert trustee, prepared a formal statement of objectives and development conditions for geographic membership in the medical center. The statement served as the basis for the hospital's lease and reflected the terms of Kurtis Froedtert's will.

Essentially Froedtert Hospital's autonomy as a freestanding, general, acute care, nonsectarian hospital was basic to any lease agreement. It would need 12.9 acres of land for the hospital facility along with the necessary parking area to accommodate personnel. The lease would insure that the hospital would be affiliated and staffed by medical school faculty physicians as well as private practitioners. The lease requested allocation of land by September 1, 1973. The mental health buildings of the South Unit were on the proposed Froedtert hospital site. The cost to demolish the buildings as well as the timetable to make the land available to Froedtert would become one of many issues to be negotiated in Froedtert's lease.

The lease not only had to be acceptable to the hospital and County officials, it was also subject to approval by the Circuit Court. The Froedtert Memorial Lutheran Hospital Trust was owned and managed by the trustees. Court action was required to release trust funds to the Froedtert Hospital Corporation to pay for the proposed construction. On November 9, 1972, Froedtert officials submitted their lease requirements to County officials. It would take nearly four years of negotiations before the Froedtert lease was signed in January 1976. A long and difficult road lay ahead. Attorney Bradley recalled the days of tedium in the lease negotiations:

> I never had the sense that there was a feeling of urgency on the part of the County. This was a real departure for them to really talk about giving a long lease for the Institutions Grounds, which they regarded as a precious jewel. I think the County was trying to be responsible in protecting the public trust in this choice piece of real estate. I don't think there was any precedent with these long term-leases where they were giving up a kind of control.

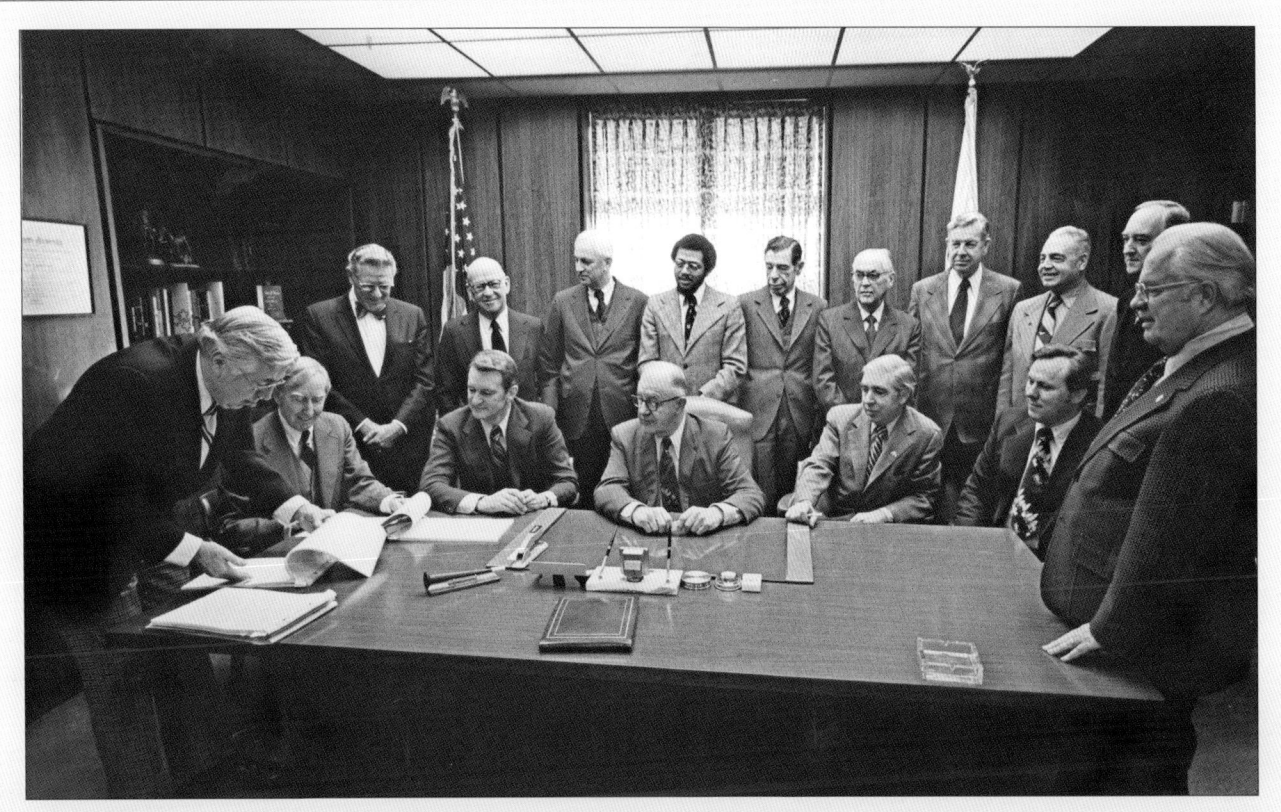

It wasn't until January 1976 that County and Froedtert officials finally signed the lease for the new hospital.

Back row: Rudolph Schoenecker, executive secretary, Greater Milwaukee Committee (GMC); Joseph Rapkin, Froedtert trustee; Wayne Roper, Froedtert legal counsel; County Supervisor Terrence Pitts; Robert Stevenson, GMC; Delbert Jacobus, Milwaukee Regional Medical Center (MRMC) board chairman; Elmer Behrens and Reginald Siebert, Froedtert board members; and Ernest Phillips, MCW board member.

Front row: County Corporation Counsel James O'Donnell; Richard Vogt, Froedtert board chairman; Dean Roe, Froedtert Hospital president; William Jahn, Froedtert board member; Milwaukee County Board Chairman William O'Donnell; Milwaukee County Clerk Thomas Zablocki; and Milwaukee County Executive John Doyne.

Bradley felt that County officials, working with private agencies on leases for public land, created some caution that added to the long delays:

> My feelings were that the Medical College, with its long relationship with the County, was not as concerned about the terms of the lease as were the Froedtert representatives. Froedtert did not have a history of working with the County. But it was going to put $20 million plus bonds into the hospital. So we felt that we had to be sure we were really going to have a long-term ongoing loyalty to Froedtert on practical business terms. Froedtert representatives felt that the patterns of the Medical College lease were not adequate to protect Froedtert's tenancy at the center. So we strengthened the lease for Froedtert and for the other private tenants as well. There were a number of clauses in the County's lease —standard in most leases—but there were clauses not covered or were not adequate for the Froedtert lease and, therefore, it took a long time to negotiate.

Froedtert's initial proposal for a one-hundred-year lease suffered a direct rebuff by the County Board's Health Committee. The Medical School and Curative leases were for fifty years, and Doyne wanted uniform lease agreements. "Bill Jahn, Froedtert's chairman, asked me to work with the negotiating team on the lease that he felt would be ready for signatures within a few weeks," Attorney Wayne Roper recalled with a smile. "The assignment was underestimated by a few years." Roper's short assignment became a permanent one. He would represent Froedtert in the lease negotiations that would take four years to finalize. He also led the battles for the hospital's rights and positions in a number of other legal skirmishes that were unforeseen at the time of the lease negotiations. Roper remained as the hospital's legal counsel for more than two decades.

The bureaucratic process played no small role in the negotiating marathon. Bradley remembers that there would be several weeks between meetings. Numerous meetings were required by supervisors and staff to review lease clauses.

While James O'Donnell, as County corporation counsel, did most of the negotiating, he did not have authority. He had to submit any changes or amendments to the Health Committee for review and approval. The Health Committee often modified issues despite negotiated agreement by both parties. This meant that negotiators would have to readdress an area that had already been explored at great length.

The location of each of the private facilities on the campus generally followed the outline developed in the master plan of 1971. Froedtert Hospital's site was five hundred to six hundred feet west of Milwaukee County General Hospital. The

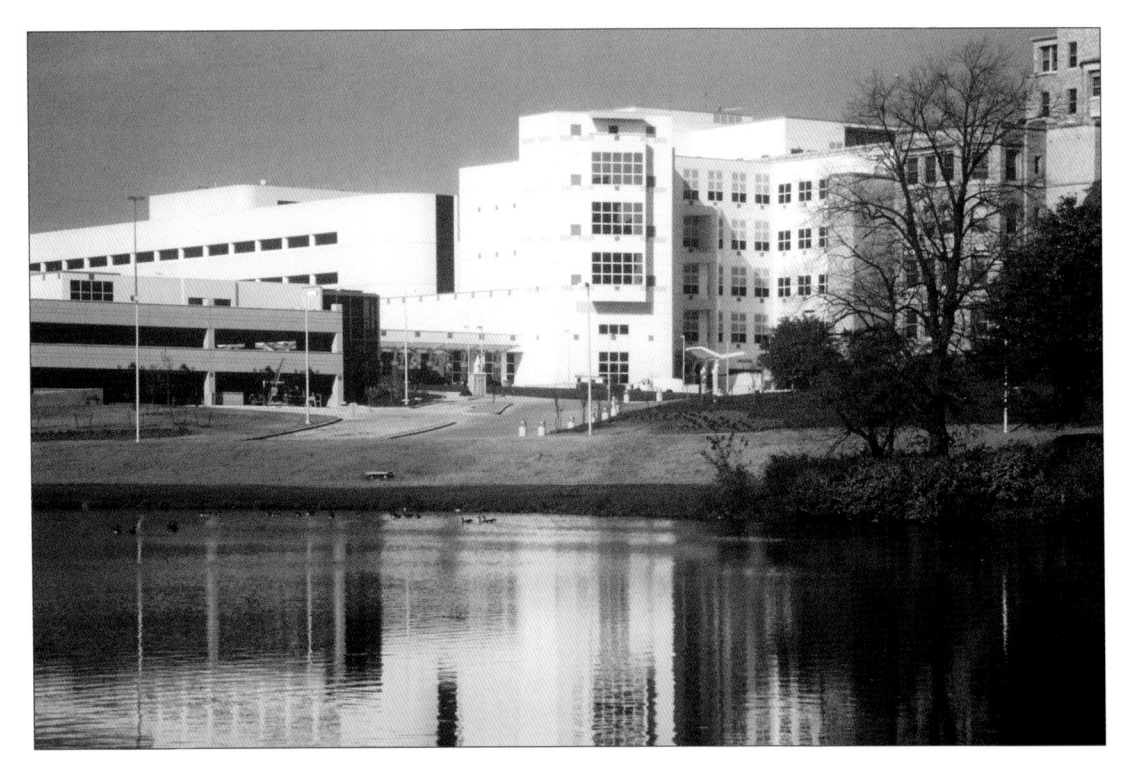

Ironically, while it took years for the shared services facility (known as the Connector or Bridge Building) to be built, it still stands today as the lower floors of the East Clinics building.

open space between County General and the Froedtert site was to be the location of a proposed shared service structure that would physically link both hospitals and serve as a gateway for patients. The shared service facility's plan and programs included laboratory, radiology, surgery, outpatient clinics, and other services.

The County's proposal and financial ability to construct the shared service or ambulatory care facility, also known as the Bridge Building, directly affected Froedtert Hospital planning. It became a major concern in the Froedtert lease negotiations. Shared use of technology in the building directly affected functional and architectural planning for Froedtert. Lease terms would have to include conditions of how both hospitals would utilize and pay for these services. There were a number of governmental hurdles to be cleared by officials of both hospitals if the shared service facility was to be constructed. Under the Comprehensive Health Planning Act, the shared service facility would have to be approved by the local planning agency, the County Board, the State Division of Health Policy and Planning, and the Wauwatosa Common Council. At best, gaining these approvals was a fifty-fifty gamble. Froedtert officials also sought reaffirmation of the County Board's role as a true and sharing partner in the medical center. ■

Chapter 17

Medical School Signs Lease

The Medical College of Wisconsin erased all doubt about its commitment to locate on the County Grounds by signing its lease on January 12, 1973. At the same time, the County Board of Supervisors ended four years of silence by voting to support the principle of a medical center. County Executive Doyne was elated with the Medical College lease and the County Board support of the medical center. But he underestimated the jousting that would take place between the private members of the medical center and the Health and Finance Committees of the County Board. The arguments would center on an equitable cost-sharing formula agreeable to all parties and contention on other issues that would delay agreement among all parties.

The medical school's signing of its lease energized action on a number of fronts. The school requested $4 million in state funding to subsidize tuition for Wisconsin residents enrolled at the Medical College of Wisconsin, the difference between tuition at the University of Wisconsin Medical School and that of the Medical College.

The planning agency approved the campus site of the Medical College Basic Science structure and the Eye Institute. This latter structure was to be connected to the County Hospital.

Lease negotiations for the other private agencies seeking a place on the County Institutions Grounds were not without days and months of frustration. The critical issue for all private members was the need for an ordinance that would define governance of the medical center and a formula for sharing expenses among all the center facilities.

However, by mid-March of 1973, a cost-sharing formula was established by a special committee of the County Board. The formula was based on occupied building space. The County's campus buildings, including the North and South Units of the Mental Health Complex, had more occupied building space than the total square footage proposed for the private members of the center. Under this formula, the County would incur 60-70 percent of the center's operating costs for walks, tunnels, landscaping, street lighting, fire and police protection, and traffic control.

70

An arbitrary decision by County officials requesting private members to share more than $590,000 in consulting and road improvements costs led to an ultimatum issued by the Medical Center Council on April 25, 1973. An angry and frustrated Medical Center Council told County officials that if problems between the County and the Council were not resolved within a 30-60 day period, some members would withdraw from locating at the center. It was imperative for the County Board and the Council to agree on governance of medical center planning.

A new cost-sharing ordinance was proposed by the Health Committee in early July. The formula called for half of any medical center expense to be split according to the square feet of building space occupied by each medical center member. To determine the share for paying the remainder of any medical center expenses, the value of the buildings would be used. Adding building value as a feature of shared cost worked to the County's benefit. Many of the buildings on the County Institutions Grounds were decades old, and some were scheduled for eventual demolition. The value of these older buildings was nominal at best. Under this revised formula, private institutions on the campus faced an additional $7.5 million in costs. Froedtert's share under this proposal would add $1 million to the hospital's construction costs.

The proposed ordinance also gave Milwaukee County the power to decide what shared services would be provided to medical center members. For example, the County could arbitrarily decide to build a roadway or improve some other aspect of the grounds. Private members would have to share the costs whether or not they agreed with the decisions. The full County Board approved the cost-sharing ordinance in mid-July of 1973. Reaction to the approved cost-sharing ordinance was predictable. The private members were incensed.

The Froedtert, Curative, and Blood Center Boards began looking at the Veterans Administration Hospital site in West Milwaukee (Wood). Meetings were held in Washington, D.C., with top officials of the Veterans Administration regarding the possibility of locating the medical center on the VA grounds. Despite its signed lease, officials of the medical school now began to consider the possibility of building its Basic Science building on the VA property. The private members retained an architectural firm to undertake a preliminary feasibility study and conceptual plan for the VA site. The standoff on cost sharing and shared governance and the search for an alternate site now seriously threatened construction of a medical center on the County Grounds. For County officials it was a startling wakeup call.

Concerned about the unraveling of the medical center on the County

Grounds, eight County supervisors introduced a resolution calling for another look at the ordinance that would define the manner in which common costs would be shared. Six months after the Medical College signed its lease, it was clear a jump start was needed to get the whole issue of governance and cost sharing resolved. ■

Chapter 18

One Crisis after Another

Lease negotiations and planning were assigned to the County Board of Public Welfare in 1973. Some critics viewed the Board of Public Welfare as a "board of directors" for the County Institutions, creating undue County power and influence. Since the Welfare Board's decisions were only advisory, final action by the Health Committee and the full County Board was required. That put the County Board in full control of medical center development. It was a point of frustration for the private members, who had waited for months to obtain acceptable terms from the Health Committee. Some of the County supervisors feared that the Welfare Board's role would usurp their control over the center's development.

While there was progress, a number of problems needed resolution before any shovels went into the ground. Froedtert had specific needs that delayed signing a lease for another two years. Froedtert refused to sign a lease until the County Board committed funds for planning and construction of the ambulatory care facility that would provide a physical link between the two hospitals and house shared services for both. The issue of the County's commitment to an ambulatory care facility was a major planning concern. If the ambulatory care structure was going to provide radiology, laboratory, and outpatient clinics to be shared by both hospitals, it would have a major impact on architectural plans and construction costs for Froedtert. Should the County back off on a commitment to construct the shared service facility, Froedtert's plans would have to include high-cost services in its new facility.

All of these issues dragged on through the early months of 1974, and a move to the Veterans Administration site began to look more promising. The engineering consultants retained by the private agencies reported that a forty-acre site at the Veterans Hospital would be suitable for all medical center facilities. Another positive factor in the decision to move to the VA site was the easy access to power, sewer, and water utilities. Representatives of the four private healthcare units had engineers look at the environmental impact as a second and important phase of planning a move to the VA medical center from the County Grounds. By March 11, 1974, the four private members announced that they were ending negotiations with the County and would seek another location after eight frustrating years of planning and negotiating for the County Grounds locale.

County Board Chairman Richard Nowakowski jumped into the breach and suggested that the County government build the Medical College's Basic Science building and lease it back over forty-five years. The proposal seemed to have some merit.

Nowakowski's offer to the Medical College was viewed by some as an attempt to split it from the other private members of the proposed medical center. Medical College Dean Kerrigan was keenly aware that hidden within an offer of this dimension were potential problems of control for programs and future school expansions if County funds were used to build the school. Nowakowski saw value in retaining the long-standing relationship between the medical school and County Hospital, since the school's faculty physicians administered the highest quality of care for the County's patients. He also knew that political control could be maintained through the County Board of Welfare.

The *Milwaukee Journal* in a March 13, 1974, editorial summed up the somewhat chaotic situation:

County's Medical Center Fiasco

Milwaukee County blew it. Chances of having the proposed Regional Medical Center where it logically belongs – on County Institutions grounds – appears dead. Center members have ceased negotiations with the County and plan to locate elsewhere.

It is a case of politics played out against the public interest under the guise of protecting the public interest. The County Board, despite the prospect of acquiring a hundred million dollars' worth of property and immeasurable benefit in terms of service and prestige, has aced itself out.

A basic impediment to resolving conflicts may have been inherent in asking a political body, without sufficient background, to settle the complex questions the center raised. Deep philosophical difference – the county's determination to control and private members' insistence on full partnership – may have precluded agreement from the start. It was a case of a legislative body trying to be an administrator.

The editorial concluded:

A new site could be agreed upon within a month. That is encouraging. However disappointing the abandonment of the county site is, it is now time to move the center off the drawing board.

At the courthouse, officials scrambled to save the day. Chairman Nowakowski scheduled a meeting that included County Executive Doyne and Supervisors Pitts and O'Donnell, along with representatives of the four private medical center members. Dr. Kerrigan made it clear to Nowakowski that the meeting was not going to be another negotiating session. He informed Nowakowski that he and the other private representatives would listen to the County officials and report to their respective boards. Nowakowski asked Medical College officials to resume negotiations and create a master lease that would serve the three private members of the medical center. The major problem was the feeling that the County was unwilling to give autonomy to the private members locating on the County Grounds. While the private representatives agreed to bring the Nowakowski proposal to their respective boards, they did not hold out hope for approval.

The dim prospects for agreement on Nowakowski's proposal ignited another effort to reopen negotiations in mid-March of 1974. A unanimous County Board resolution directed the corporation counsel to work out a master lease with the Medical College to serve as a pattern for lease agreements for the private agencies. An interesting addendum was included in the resolution: Approved leases for the private members would enable each to acquire additional land without going back through the County Board for approval. The land could be granted by the Board of Public Welfare. The resolution was enticing, but the private members continued working toward a move to the VA site.

The Medical College Executive Committee agreed to resume negotiations. Attorneys Michael Bolger, the medical school counsel, and Robert Russell, the County's corporation counsel, held marathon negotiating sessions and in mid-April fashioned a master lease that the County Board approved. The Medical Center master lease included supplemental agreements to meet the requirements of the Blood Center, Curative, and Froedtert. However, County Board approval was needed for each supplemental agreement. Curative and Blood Center agreements were approved 23-1 by the County Board.

Froedtert's approval was another story. The 19-5 vote on that lease indicated that Froedtert was viewed as a competitive threat to County General. In its supplemental agreement, Froedtert gave the County an additional year to relocate patients and personnel in the South Division mental health buildings that were on the proposed site for the new hospital. Giving the County this extra time was a concession as well as a gamble. In a year's time, the cost of financing the hospital as well as price increases in materials and equipment could affect the construction costs of Froedtert Hospital.

Under the newly crafted master lease, the County gave up much of the control. The Medical Center Council would oversee the policies and programs of the center. This was a landmark decision.

The leases defined the area and amount of land that each private member would occupy, the dates by which the premises must be cleared, the uses to which the sites must be confined, and other conditions relative to each of the agencies. Froedtert's Board of Directors approved the lease on April 24, 1974. To insure that the lease agreement did not violate the terms of Kurtis Froedtert's will, the trustees petitioned the court for authorization to enter into a lease. Froedtert's attorney, Wayne Roper, was successful in gaining court approval to release construction funds from the Kurtis Froedtert Trust. Judge William J. Shaughnessy gave that authorization on May 6, 1974. It would appear that the all-clear signal had sounded for the start of facility construction. Such was not the case. A number of troublesome situations arose to cause further delays.

The Medical College was facing a tight deadline to obtain a $20 million guaranteed federal loan; the legislation for this loan program would end on June 30. In mid-June, the four private members of the Medical Center stated they would not sign their leases until the County Welfare Board approved the Ambulatory Care Agreement, the site surveys for each private facility were completed, and agreement was reached on the road network of the center.

This wall of solidarity by the four private members on lease signing began to weaken. The long delays in negotiations escalated building costs and forced the Curative Board to sign its lease in mid-July. The remaining private members agreed to hold off on signing until the medical school financing was assured and the other agreements were reached. This mutual pact among the remaining private members was also on shaky ground.

The school's precarious status and the uncertainties of the medical center development forced the August 6 announcement that the Milwaukee Blood Center would search for another site. The loss of the Blood Center as a geographic member was viewed as a major disappointment. Three days later, the medical school announced that it would sign its lease in a show of "good faith" despite its construction financing problem. By the end of August 1974, the County Board approved the medical school's signed lease.

The good faith gesture by the medical school was confirmed by a series of events in the next few months. The community fundraising drive was revived as the Medical College of Wisconsin began piecing together private and public financing. The drive had been halted in 1972 because of financial difficulties and delays in getting a building site approved on the County Grounds. The goal was to raise $18 million.

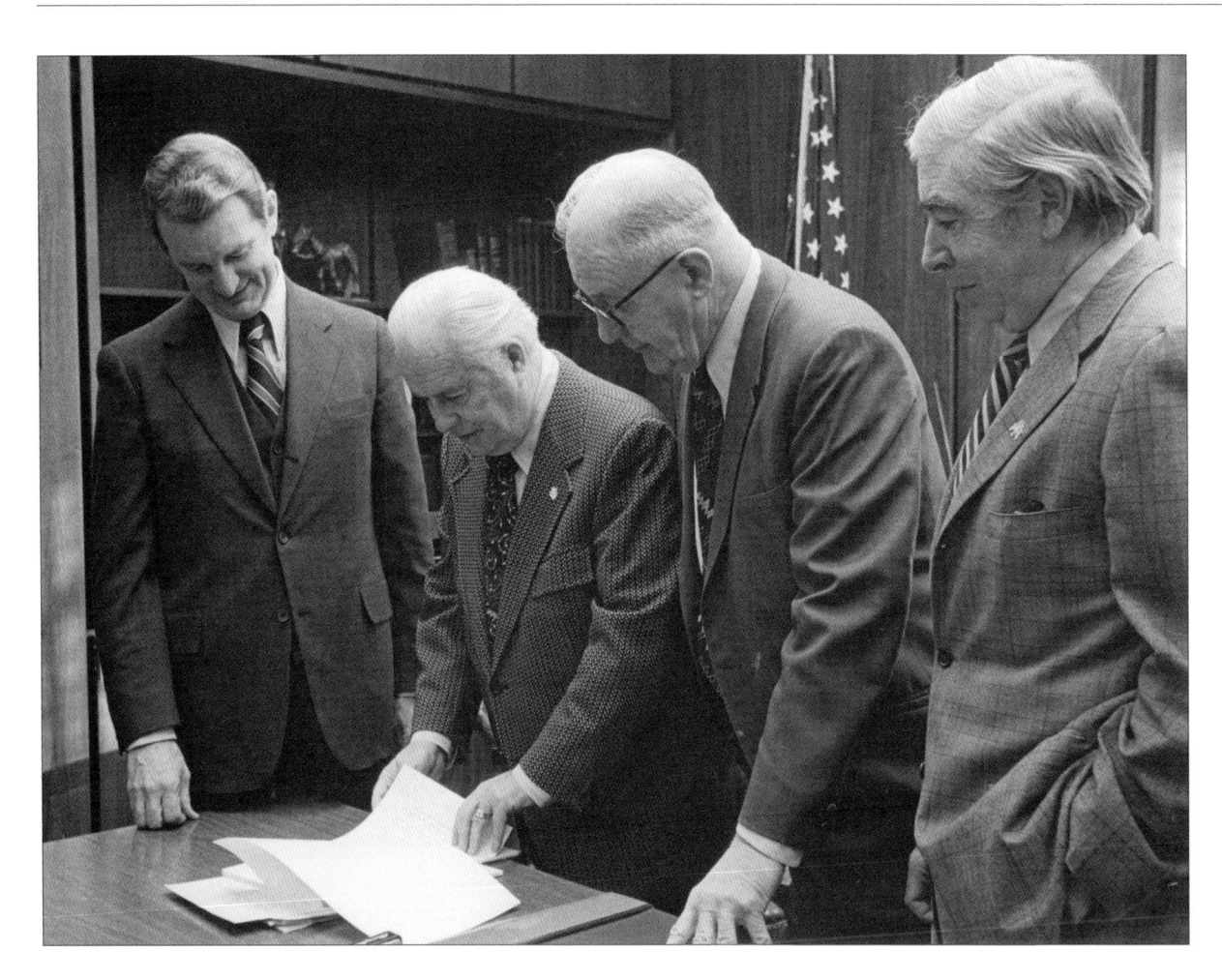

In the opening days of 1975, Froedtert negotiators sought an agreement with the County on the ambulatory care facility. The lease negotiations would continue to drag on through the spring and mid-summer months.

County Board negotiators re-ignited the moribund lease negotiations by seeking answers to sixteen separate issues or questions. The most important question included Froedtert's position allowing access to Froedtert's clinical services by all patients coming to the medical center. Other major items included financial support of teaching and research at the Medical College and protection of County employees who would transfer with the services that would be moved to Froedtert. Roe and the Froedtert negotiators felt that the requests would not be a problem, but lease negotiations dragged

Finally, in January 1976 the lease is signed. Left to right: Froedtert Hospital President Dean Roe, County Executive John Doyne, Froedtert Hospital Board Vice President William Jahn, and Milwaukee County Board President William O'Donnell look over the document.

on through late fall and into the winter months.

While things were at an impasse with Froedtert's lease during 1975, substantial progress was made in the medical school's quest for financing and construction of its Basic Science building. The catalyst for this storm of activity was David Carley, who had become the Medical College's first lay president in February 1975. By mid-summer he engineered assurances of a $7 million federal grant, $8 million from the state, and a $10 million loan from the State Investment Board. This base of public funding served as a catalyst for the private fund drive to reach the $42 million needed for construction of the school's Basic Science building. Meanwhile the Froedtert lease struggle went on. At the end of 1975, there were no signatures affixed. In fact, it wasn't until the beginning of the next year that Froedtert and County officials would sign a lease. ∎

Chapter 19

Need for a Medical Center?

In 1976, the Comprehensive Health Planning Agency of Southeastern Wisconsin (CHPASEW) continued to question the need for Froedtert Hospital in light of the surplus of hospital beds. The health planning agency questioned the size and services of the proposed ambulatory care facility. They saw a need for wide distribution of outpatient services throughout the city rather than at a centrally located service, and concerns were expressed about the educational aspects of the medical center. CHPASEW members feared that too many specialist and sub-specialist physicians would be trained when primary care doctors were needed. Private hospital representatives in the agency viewed the medical center as direct competition with their own facilities.

The health planning agency also questioned the possible move of Children's Hospital to the County Grounds, away from the central city. Agency staff felt that the County should contract with existing hospitals for care of the mentally ill rather than build new facilities on the County Grounds.

Dr. Walter Rattan, then president of the CHPASEW, suggested that Froedtert Trust funds be used to purchase County General Hospital or be given directly to either the Medical College or Children's Hospital for construction of their facilities. These public expressions from the planning agency appeared presumptuous to medical center officials. Plans for Froedtert and Children's hospitals and for the County's mental health facility had not yet been submitted to the agency. The atmosphere was a bit foreboding.

The Medical Center Council responded to CHPASEW's troubling observations. The council suggested that Milwaukee County General, Froedtert, and Children's hospitals be classified as "statewide facilities," similar to the status enjoyed by the University of Wisconsin Hospital in Madison. Their strategy was to remove medical center facilities from a purely local or regional status and gain a more favorable position with the planning agency. The issue of more than one thousand excess hospital beds in the area continued to be key in the approval process.

The Children's Hospital announcement to renovate its downtown facility and the controversy over the need to build Froedtert Hospital brought about another surprising and public response from the health planners. CHPASEW officials thought that Children's could be constructed as a wing of the proposed Froedtert facility. Children's administration said that autonomy was necessary for their operation and that merging with a general hospital made it difficult to meet the needs of the pediatric patient. ■

Chapter 20

The Bumpy Road to Approval

After twenty-five years of wrangling, Froedtert Hospital filed a notice of intent with the State Division of Health Policy and Planning in early June 1976. The formal, one-hundred-page application was submitted to the planners on August 26. Under federal law, area and state planning staffs had sixty days to study and render a decision on the application. The deadline for a decision was October 26. A timely approval meant that groundbreaking for the new hospital could be scheduled within a year. The deadline turned out to be a major problem for the planners and Froedtert officials.

The application squarely faced the issue of excess beds. Froedtert and County General hospitals agreed to divide services and reduce the total number of beds on the campus. This move was made to soften the outcry of surplus beds by the planning staff. The number of beds in the two hospitals would total 720: Froedtert would be a 300-bed facility and County General would have 420 beds.

The announcement of Froedtert's application brought immediate response from local hospital officials. The principal fear of city and suburban hospitals was loss of patients. Others challenged Froedtert's role as an advanced teaching hospital. Some officials said that recent additions to community hospitals had established tertiary services—there was no need to build any more. Medical school officials countered this position and emphasized the efficiencies in research, teaching, and patient care through accessible tertiary service in one location. The two nationally known consultants retained earlier by the Froedtert trustees had criticized the widely separated clinical teaching sites in Milwaukee.

The reaction to Froedtert's application and to the Milwaukee Regional Medical Center itself became a widely discussed matter by healthcare officials, community leaders, and, to a lesser degree, the general public. Newspapers wrote several articles on increased hospital and healthcare costs. The stories did not bolster Froedtert's cause. One follow-up story questioned the need for County General Hospital, since Medicare and Medicaid patients could now choose any hospital for care at less expense to taxpayers. The barrage of comment and criticism created openly antagonistic attitudes toward Froedtert Hospital and the whole idea of an academic medical center.

As the October deadline approached, health planners asked for more time to review the application. The Executive Committee of the recently renamed Southeastern Wisconsin Health Systems Agency (SEWHSA) indicated that a thorough review of the application might take until the end of the year—far beyond the sixty-day review limit and the October 26 deadline. Planning staff members said that numerous questions about the application needed to be answered by Froedtert officials. Roe had already responded to additional questions from the planning agency and submitted these on September 27. There were indications from unnamed planning staff that approval might be denied if the agency had to decide on the application by the October 26 deadline.

Froedtert's Board agreed to extend the deadline for fifty days, but the planning staff turned down the offer. What the planning agency really wanted was a withdrawal of the application filed on August 27, 1976. The planners wanted Froedtert to re-submit its application based on the September 27 date on which they had received additional requested information from Froedtert. That way, the planners could have a renewed sixty-day time span to review the application.

That strategy drew considerable interest from the editorial board of the *Milwaukee Journal*. An editorial on October 15, 1976, castigated the planners and asked burning questions about the approval process for Froedtert:

Get Ahead on Froedtert

Area health planners are behaving strangely on the application of Froedtert Memorial Lutheran Hospital for approval to build on County Institutions grounds. Undoubtedly they are being subjected to strong political pressures, most of which would have them turn down Froedtert. But the Health Policy Planning Council and Area Health Systems Agency are supposed to be objective and independent decision makers. The dance they are presently doing, first asking to postpone their decision and then turning down Froedtert's offer of an extension of the legal deadline, leads to the suspicion that their strings are being pulled by considerations other than the merit of the application itself.

The law provides that applications such as Froedtert's be decided in two months, to shield applicants from long delays that increase their costs. It is doubtful whether any application has been more thoroughly prepared and fully presented. Two weeks after it was submitted planners had further questions, relayed to Froedtert in a letter that did not arrive for several weeks. Then, still later, more questions arose. Planners asked Froedtert to withdraw the original application and let its September 27th information serve as a new one – with a new deadline. This was accompanied by a thinly veiled threat that if Froedtert refused, its application was likely to be rejected. Then when Froedtert, though not required to do so, offered a 50 day delay, it was rejected. An explanation is due.

Is it possible that planners intend to turn down Froedtert first time around in order to appease those community hospitals, over-bedded and over-equipped that perceive a threat in still more beds? Is it possible that some time in the months ahead planners will approve Froedtert as part of a sweeping plan to eliminate excess beds throughout the area, and that the heat would then fall on Froedtert rather than the state planners? Is it possible that the University of Wisconsin Hospitals feels so threatened by the medical center in Milwaukee, and the possibility of losing patients to it, that the Madison group would try to scuttle the new center by pressuring for a Froedtert rejection?

Froedtert has acted in good faith in submitting its application, providing answers as requested and offering to extend the deadline. Health planners are right to be concerned about adding hospital beds but would be wrong to use bed count alone as justification for denying Froedtert's application. That hospital's location, purpose and treatment would not duplicate existing services. As a key component of the Medical College and the medical center, Froedtert would provide a service not possible from six beds here and a dozen there in general hospitals scattered around the community. Further, the federal and state grants that are enabling the college to build were based on the school's access to the teaching facility that Froedtert and County General Hospitals would provide. It is unthinkable that health planners, regardless of political pressures, would ignore so vital a public interest as that served by giving Froedtert approval to go ahead. It is, after all, the public interest that health planners are committed to serve.

The editorial appeared on the same day that state planning and Froedtert officials reached a compromise to allow the state until December 15, and possibly longer, to make a final decision on the application. In turn, Froedtert officials agreed to provide any additional information by November 15. The responses would be part of the formal application. Under the agreement, Froedtert would not have to withdraw any part of its application and the state would get from four to six additional weeks to consider it. State health planners then asked to have until January 4, 1977, to make their decision. Public meetings were scheduled for the first week in December.

Two weeks after agreement was reached with state and area planners, Froedtert and Lutheran hospitals disclosed plans to merge. The announcement, on November 2, 1976, came amid local hospital opposition to Froedtert's construction. The proposed merger meant that Froedtert would plan its 300-bed hospital with the possibility that Lutheran would decrease its 440 beds by 166 beds over three years while the new hospital was under construction.

In prior months, some of the most direct and somewhat critical comments on Froedtert and the medical center were voiced by Donald Mundt, Lutheran Hospital Board chairman and a vice-president of Northwestern Mutual Insurance Company. His comments centered on the efficient use of the community's health resources. He felt the community had to seek a plan through which the medical center could grow without adding excess hospital beds. Mundt launched the idea of a merger in preliminary meetings with the boards of Lutheran and Froedtert. Under the plan, the merged institution would operate at Lutheran Hospital while Froedtert was under construction.

Roe recalled:

> The purpose behind the merger was that Froedtert gained a downtown location that was financially sound and had a rich tradition and history. Lutheran gained a relationship with an ongoing entity that had a future in an academic setting. Both would be strengthened through the merger. You would have a single entity, Froedtert Memorial Lutheran Hospital, a teaching facility at the medical center as well as a community hospital downtown.

There were a number of benefits to the merger, not the least of which was a favorable review of Froedtert's application by health planners. It would not add beds. The start-up costs for Froedtert would be reduced and, finally, using the assets of the financially strong Lutheran Hospital would assure the Medical College of a new teaching hospital for its expanding student enrollment.

Other benefits included the use of a vacated Lutheran Hospital by Children's or Deaconess hospitals, purchase by Marquette University, or as a downtown medical center for Milwaukee County. The widely heralded idea of a merger drew interest from the area and state planners. In time, the concept of merging hospitals became the health planners' hole card. The health planners played it to the hilt.

While the hospital merger captured the headlines, SEWHSA staff continued its review of Froedtert's application and posed more than eighty additional questions that required responses by the November 15 date. There was no opposition to Froedtert's application at a public hearing that drew only fourteen people. At the hearing, a representative from Deaconess suggested that Lutheran Hospital close its acute care beds if the merged institution came about. The idea would reduce the surplus bed count and Deaconess would stand alone in the neighborhood as an adult acute care facility.

In a masterpiece of bad timing, the staff of SEWHSA released a revised report on Froedtert's application. The report was issued—and published—just eight days before the area planning agency was to announce its decision on Froedtert's application to build. Replies to more than eighty questions the agency asked of Froedtert officials were included in the report that listed more disadvantages than advantages for Froedtert's application.

The agency report said Froedtert would drain $66 million in patient revenue from area hospitals in the first three years of its operation. Construction would add to the excess beds. The agency estimated that Froedtert would cost the public between $18 million and $33 million in the first three years of operation that would be reflected in higher patient bills. The planning agency acknowledged and recognized Froedtert Hospital's role as a teaching facility to train and retain doctors for the state and the area. It acknowledged that the planned sub-specialty services would attract needed specialists to the area. But there were few other positive responses to Froedtert's application. The report was anything but encouraging.

However, the picture brightened considerably on December 8. The health planning agency's Facilities Review Committee approved Froedtert's application in a 13-5 vote. The four-hour meeting was highlighted by the support of Froedtert's application by County Supervisor Pitts. He pushed for Froedtert's approval as a needed facility for the medical school and indicated that without Froedtert's presence at the medical center, county taxpayers would have to come up with money for health facilities. His presentation of the Froedtert position was a key element in the 13-5 vote. At this point it looked as though final approval would be given at the SEWHSA Executive Committee meeting, scheduled for December 10, 1976. ■

Chapter 21

All Tied Up

The meeting of the Southeastern Wisconsin Health Systems Agency (SEWHSA) Executive Committee was not without its political sideshow. Donovan Riley, vice president of the Medical College and a member of the SEWHSA Executive Committee, was declared ineligible to vote since the school and Froedtert were in a formal teaching agreement. A similar move was made to remove Supervisor Pitts, chairman of the County Board's Health Committee. Pitts was considered a Froedtert proponent. He survived the motion to remove him from the vote. After nearly two hours of debate and political maneuvering, the vote ended in a tie. The disqualification of Riley, who would have voted for approval, proved to be crucial. The Froedtert application would go to the state Division of Health Policy and Planning in Madison without recommendation. It was devastating news for Froedtert and medical center officials.

While the tie vote appeared to negate years of planning and negotiating, it actually put the application in the hands of Ralph Andreano, administrator of the State Division of Health Policy and Planning. The final decision would be up to him. His December 31 deadline was just twenty-one days away.

On the same day that SEWHSA cast its 9-9 vote, representatives of Deaconess and Lutheran hospitals reopened earlier discussions regarding a three-way affiliation. The idea was to have Deaconess form an alliance with Lutheran and then have Lutheran consolidate with Froedtert. A reduction in hospital beds was envisioned through the close working relationship of the three hospitals.

Froedtert's application was now in the hands of Ralph Andreano. Within two weeks, Andreano let it be known that the plans and application for Froedtert Hospital would be rejected unless there was a firm agreement from Froedtert officials to consolidate with one or more hospitals. Suddenly the pressure shifted from Madison back to Milwaukee. Froedtert and Lutheran officials reacted quickly, telling Andreano that the merger was virtually accomplished. Andreano had two days to make a decision. He said if Froedtert did not ask for an extension or indicate that it would merge with Lutheran and possibly Deaconess, he would "drop the bomb," as the *Milwaukee Sentinel* reported on December 26, 1976. That symbolic warhead would most assuredly obliterate the proposed Froedtert Hospital.

Roe was confident that the merger agreement could be reached, although he was concerned that the merger might require a planning agency review and jeopardize the current building plans. Andreano indicated that if he had evidence in writing of an agreement between Froedtert and Lutheran, he would make a quick decision.

Clearly Andreano was pushing for a three-hospital merger, because he thought it would reduce the inefficiencies and costs of Milwaukee's hospital system. He even suggested that Froedtert management move into Lutheran Hospital at North 22nd Street and Kilbourn Avenue while Froedtert was being built. Upon completion of Froedtert, the newly formed Lutheran-Froedtert corporation would move to the new facility at the medical center. Deaconess would then move from its structure on North 19th Street to the Lutheran facility. The old Deaconess building could then be used as an outpatient clinic for the central city. The merger card that Andreano was playing was the only power he had to affect the surplus beds in Milwaukee hospitals. Once Froedtert's plans were approved, his power to engineer substantial change was diminished.

The deadline for decisions was at hand, and the merger situation was not as settled as first believed. Roe asked state planning officials to hold off until January 5, 1977, to give Froedtert and Lutheran officials more time to work out a merger with the possibility of including Deaconess. However, there were problems to be resolved before any assurances could be given to the state planners.

On January 5, the day before the deadline, officials of Lutheran, Froedtert, and Deaconess announced a commitment-in-principle to merge. A joint merger team would be formed to continue negotiations to establish a consolidated hospital system. The merger team would plan how to consolidate Deaconess and Lutheran prior to the opening of the new Froedtert Hospital. Officials said that boards of Lutheran and Froedtert had approved a merger agreement that would be signed when the state approved the Froedtert application.

The merger announcement also called for pooling the three hospitals' assets, including the Lutheran and Deaconess buildings and land, and a $7 million trust fund from the Froedtert Hospital Trust. Roe would be the operating head of Lutheran while Froedtert was under construction. Ken Jamron, Deaconess administrator, would head the downtown center when Froedtert's building was completed.

While the announcement pleased Andreano, he said he would announce his final decision the following day. He continued to push for establishing ambulatory care services in the Deaconess building if its services moved to the Lutheran facility.

The long and arduous journey and fulfillment of Kurt Froedtert's vision was emblazoned in a bold, eight-column, front-page headline of the *Milwaukee Sentinel's* edition of January 6, 1977. Four words said it all:

State OKs Froedtert Hospital

Andreano met the deadline but imposed conditions. Froedtert must agree to reduce the new hospital's bed size from 300 to 278 and merge with Deaconess and Lutheran hospitals. He said consolidation of the three hospitals would reduce the thirteen hundred surplus beds in the area by one-third. Merging Deaconess and Lutheran would create a single, financially strong general hospital in downtown Milwaukee and improve outpatient services for central city residents.

SEWHSA needed assurance that a three-hospital merger would take place. A clause was inserted into the agreement requiring ninety days of mediation before ending any merger talks. Mediation would be done by the local planning agency, a clause that would be invoked in the months ahead. The merger of the three hospitals turned out to be a major clash of personalities and conflicting management philosophies.

Later, as a University of Wisconsin professor emeritus of economics, Andreano recalled the factors involving his decision to approve the Froedtert Hospital construction. In the quiet of his UW campus office in Madison, he reflected on those crucial days as the administrator of the Division of Health Policy and Planning. "I never felt that I wasn't going to approve Froedtert," he acknowledged. "I was trying to shape it up a little bit."

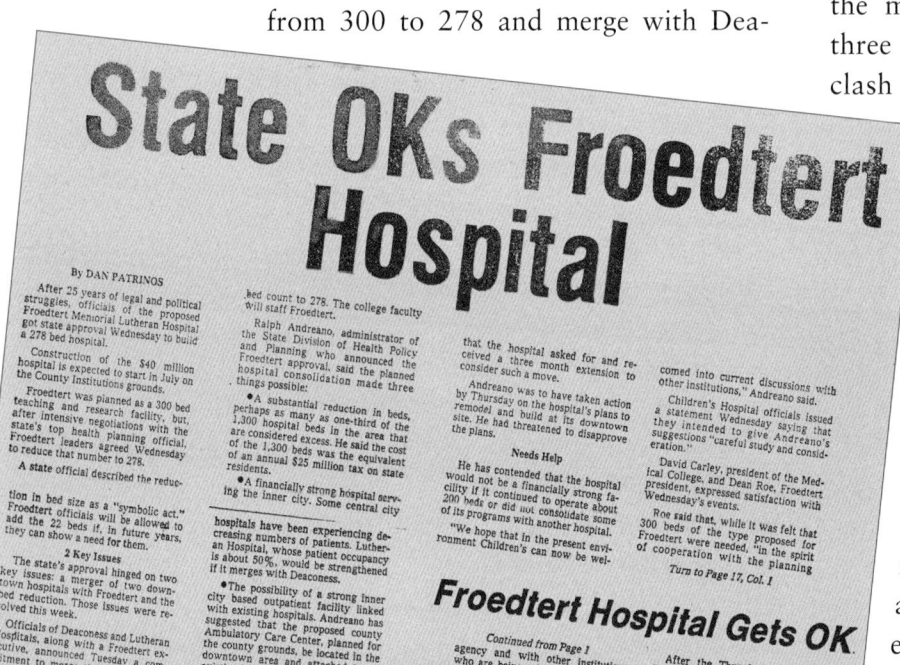

Andreano's decision centered on the Medical College and its long-term affiliation with a teaching hospital. He was concerned about the difficulties County General Hospital was experiencing at the time. The hospital had a review team looking at problems in its accounting, billing, and other management functions. These problems raised a question in Andreano's mind about County General's ability to continue a long-term role and relationship with the medical school. He recognized that the medical school had to have a viable teaching hospital affiliation in future years and that the Froedtert Hospital Trust provided a degree of long-term viability for the new hospital.

"If the Medical College was needed, then we had to have a place for them to practice, to have tertiary services, to train residents, and to recruit high quality people to teach in the medical school," he recalled. "So I linked them. Ultimately that was what I had in mind when I approved Froedtert." In the years ahead, Andreano's analysis and vision would prove to be prophetic.

The County General problems also concerned Medical College President David Carley. Three weeks after Froedtert's approval, he suggested creating an independent hospital board to run the County's medical institutions. He also said that the school would be willing to consider leasing or buying the hospital to help solve its financial problems. He added that the school did not want to get into the hospital management business.

In March 1977, the Medical College board hired a consultant to study the operations of County General Hospital and the Mental Health Center. The inefficient operation of the County Institutions, according to the Medical College, was the result of County government bureaucracy.

Andreano's charge to reduce the perceived excess beds through a three-hospital merger was viewed as possible, but not without some major problems. The three hospitals formed a merger team. It retained three different hospital consulting firms to conduct a study of the proposal: James A. Hamilton and Associates of Minneapolis; Anthony J.J. Rourke, Inc. of Harrison, New York; and Herman Smith Associates of Hinsdale, Illinois. All three were nationally recognized experts in hospital planning. The cost of the study was estimated at $100,000. Since the study would take an estimated nine months, an immediate merger was out of the question.

The conditions of the merger as part of the approval for Froedtert's construction brought about a rather startling development. With prior approval of the boards of Froedtert and Lutheran hospitals, Roe was elected president of Lutheran Hospital on February 23, 1977. His duties at Lutheran would begin March 1. He would also remain as president of Froedtert.

"Don Mundt, chairman of Lutheran's Board, had been working toward a merger with Deaconess Hospital because they were just a few blocks apart and both were struggling a bit at the time," Roe recalled. "There were enough rifts in the negotiations between Lutheran and Deaconess to dampen the prospects for a successful merger of these facilities." Negotiations on a Deaconess-Lutheran merger came to a halt. At this point, Lutheran turned its attention to a possible merger with Froedtert Hospital. Roe recalled:

> The boards of Lutheran and Froedtert were compatible and when we got together we saw some advantages for both hospitals. The medical school was willing to move some programs to help Lutheran. There was board action created to commit both hospitals to merge and papers were signed to create a single entity. However, the hospitals remained separate entities at this point. The two-hospital merger could have created a hospital system and would have been the first of its kind in the state.

Roe's dual role was viewed as a strong indication of substantial progress. Questions were raised, however. The appointment of Roe to head Lutheran was considered temporary. There was speculation that he would be made the CEO of any merged, three-hospital corporation. On the other side of the table, Deaconess officials felt that they should be considered for the leadership of a Lutheran-Deaconess merger downtown while the new Froedtert Hospital was under construction. To the Deaconess people, Roe's appointment as the Lutheran Hospital president appeared to be permanent. This raised the possibility that Lutheran held an inside position in the run for the administration of a Lutheran-Deaconess merger.

Roe now faced the formidable task of the merger as well as planning and coordinating the Froedtert Hospital construction project. A week after his appointment to head two hospitals, he named John R. Shepard as senior vice president of Froedtert. Shepard, administrator of Appleton Memorial Hospital for fifteen years, would assist in planning and overseeing the new hospital construction.

While the three-hospital merger was now in the hands of professional consulting firms, other action was taking place in a changing Milwaukee healthcare environment. In early April 1977, Children's and Deaconess hospitals signed an agreement to look at the possibilities of sharing major medical services.

Another key construction project was the ambulatory care facility that the County planned as the gateway for the two hospitals. This structure would house the medical and surgical clinics, emergency room and trauma center, and radiology and pathology services as well as operating rooms. The estimated cost of

$25 million to $42 million made it highly unlikely that county taxpayers would foot the bill. Carley told the County Board's Finance Committee that the Medical College would build it. He also told County authorities the school was not interested in managing the County's health facilities but would do so if governance changes were not made in the management structure of the institutions.

Carley's presentation to County officials was one of his last acts on behalf of the medical school. His political expertise, initiative, and vision for the medical school had brought about federal, state, local, and private financial support for a new Basic Science building on the medical center campus. He tendered his resignation but continued to serve the school as a board member. Dr. Leonard W. Cronkhite Jr., president of Children's Hospital and Medical Center of Boston, was named the school's new president, with his tenure slated to begin September 1, 1977.

Preparations for the Froedtert project went into high gear during the summer months. The County demolished the aging structures of the Mental Health Center to clear the site for the new hospital. The Froedtert Hospital Trust provided $18 million for construction and hospital start-up costs. The balance of the construction cost was financed through a City of Wauwatosa tax-free municipal bond issue of $28 million. The tax-exempt bond issue would save Froedtert Hospital about $17 million in interest over thirty years.

Negotiations for the three-hospital merger continued. The plan would have one board for the merged Deaconess and Lutheran hospitals and another for Froedtert. These two boards would be divisional boards to deal with policies. A corporate board would have responsibility for overall direction of the three merged hospitals. Members of the new corporate board would be drawn from the existing boards of Deaconess, Lutheran, and Froedtert. The commitment to a three-hospital merger was short-lived. Within three weeks, Deaconess announced its willingness to merge with Lutheran but not with Froedtert.

Deaconess justified its pull-out by declaring that its medical staff feared domination by Froedtert and the Medical College physicians. If the merger shifted hospital care to the Lutheran site, resignations from the Deaconess medical staff were predicted. It was abundantly clear that Deaconess sought to strengthen its position if a two-hospital merger came about. Deaconess officials said that a dual merger with Lutheran could effectively reduce the number of hospitals beds by two hundred. Decisions as to which of the two hospitals would close could be made at a later date. Lutheran officials held firm to a three-way merger and rejected the Deaconess plan. For months, the merger was "on again, off again." Planning officials were determined to reduce excess beds in Milwaukee. They reminded officials that consolidation of hospital services in downtown Milwaukee was a key element of the approval for Froedtert's construction.

This surprising move by Deaconess sparked a warning from Andreano. The State Division of Health administrator threatened rejection of any proposed additions or changes at the three hospitals unless the merger took place. He said he would hold the hospitals to agreements made at the time of the Froedtert approval, namely to reduce bed counts, establish outpatient services, and consolidate hospital services to benefit central city residents.

As the months passed in 1977, area and state planners were true to their threats to disapprove any applications made by any of the three hospitals involved in the mandate to merge. The regional health planning agency rejected a Deaconess proposal for a $750,000 building to house a postgraduate residency program in family practice.

Froedtert Hospital was also running into some problems in the days before groundbreaking. Detailed architectural plans and increased costs of equipment were cited as factors in a $3.8 million cost overrun that put total construction at $41 million. Because of the cost increase and Froedtert's request to increase bed capacity from the approved 278 to 285, there was a possibility that the Froedtert construction application would have to be reviewed all over again. But Andreano did not feel that a new review was necessary. The original approval allowed Froedtert to add beds if they were needed for funding the hospital construction costs. Once again, Andreano's judgment and decisiveness ruled the day. ■

Chapter 22

At Last! Groundbreaking

Despite the standstill on the hospital merger, Froedtert officials broke ground for the new hospital on a bright and sunny Wednesday morning, September 14, 1977. A proud Mary Froedtert, widow of the hospital's benefactor, turned over the first shovel of dirt to officially open construction of the $41 million facility that was her late husband's dream. Other participants wielding shiny silver shovels included: William Jahn, chairman of the Froedtert Hospital Board of Directors; Richard Vogt, Froedtert's first president and board chairman; Attorney Joseph Rapkin, Froedtert trustee; Wauwatosa

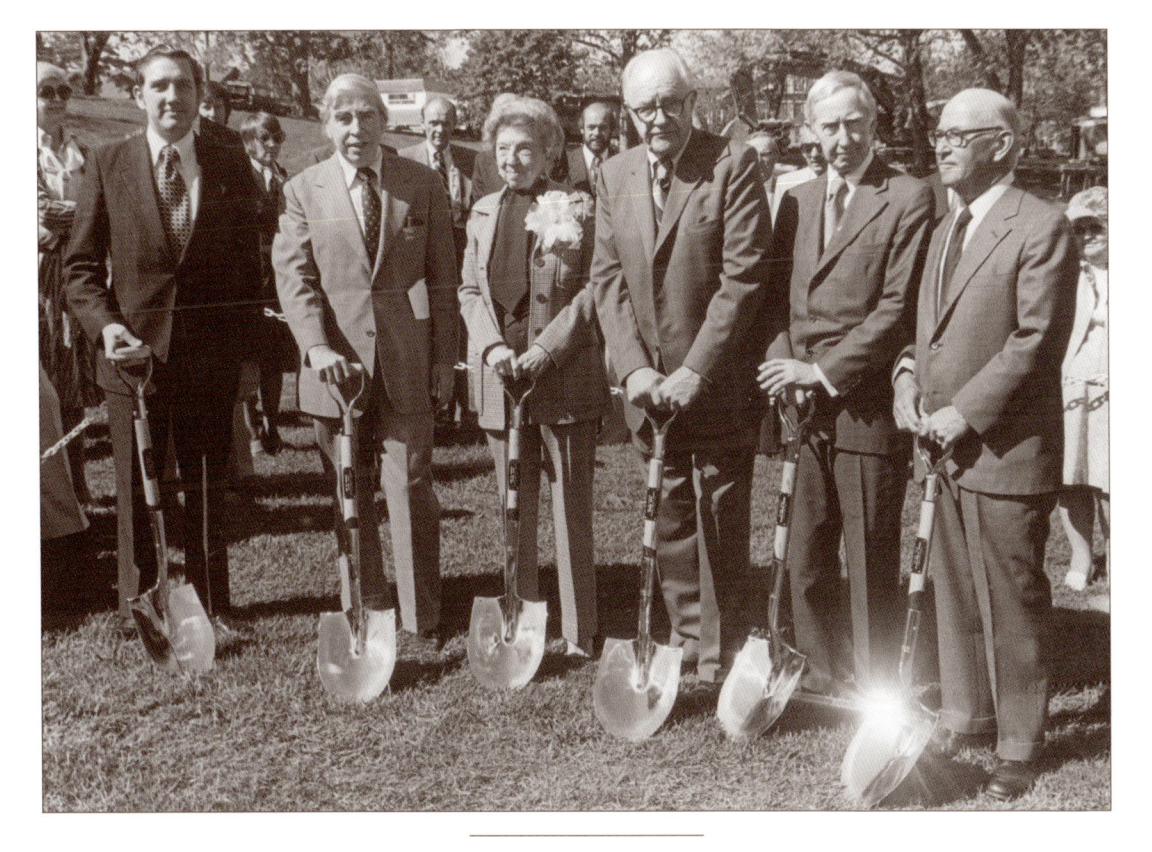

The Groundbreaking Ceremonies featured (left to right) Wauwatosa Mayor James Benz; Milwaukee County Board Chairman William O'Donnell; Kurt Froedtert's widow, Mary; Hospital Board Officers William Jahn and Richard Vogt; and Froedtert Trustee Joseph Rapkin.

Mayor James Benz; and County Board Chairman William J. O'Donnell. More than four hundred people attended the ceremony that concluded a long and sometimes torturous journey begun twenty-six years earlier.

While it was a day of smiles and satisfaction, there were problems ahead for Froedtert. There would be litigation on shared costs for a computer information system and threatened litigation with the state over a CT scanner. Questions would be raised on the ambulatory care facility and on final hospital construction costs.

Froedtert's building committee was headed by Clement Schwingle, president of American Appraisal Company. Roe recalled that Schwingle "was a key factor in every aspect of the construction project from selection of architects through detailed planning and oversight of the facility." As a board member, Schwingle worked tirelessly with his committee on all the planning details for a hospital to be like no other in Southeastern Wisconsin. Schwingle strove to insure that Froedtert would have the necessary ancillary services for patients needing specialty care as well as space for clinical research and medical education. He was committed to seeing that this hospital met and exceeded the criteria for a teaching and patient care facility. The construction site for this almost three-hundred-bed hospital of 390,000 square feet was 500 feet west of County General Hospital.

The architectural firm of Stone, Maracini, and Patterson of San Francisco was lead architect, working in conjunction with Brust-Zimmerman of Wauwatosa, now known as as Zimmerman Architectural Studios. The California architectural firm was selected because it had developed a unique building system for Veterans Administration hospitals nationally. That system included the use of interstitial space—a floor between each patient floor—that housed all heating, air conditioning, oxygen, gas and electrical, and plumbing runs. This interstitial space is high enough to accommodate work crews comfortably to make repairs or major renovations. In addition, this design creates the flexibility needed in a teaching hospital where technology and new patient service programs require frequent remodeling or renovations.

The original hospital structure, now the West Hospital, has three patient floors with twenty-eight beds in each of four quadrants, or legs, of an H-shaped structure. The large, round, exterior columns on each corner of Froedtert West house independent mechanical units for each quadrant. The separate mechanical systems enable the hospital to close one unit for renovation while the other three units on the floor remain in use. The center section of the H contains general service areas such as elevators, supply rooms, lavatories, and offices, allowing greater flexibility in moving or

Chapter 22: At Last! Groundbreaking 95

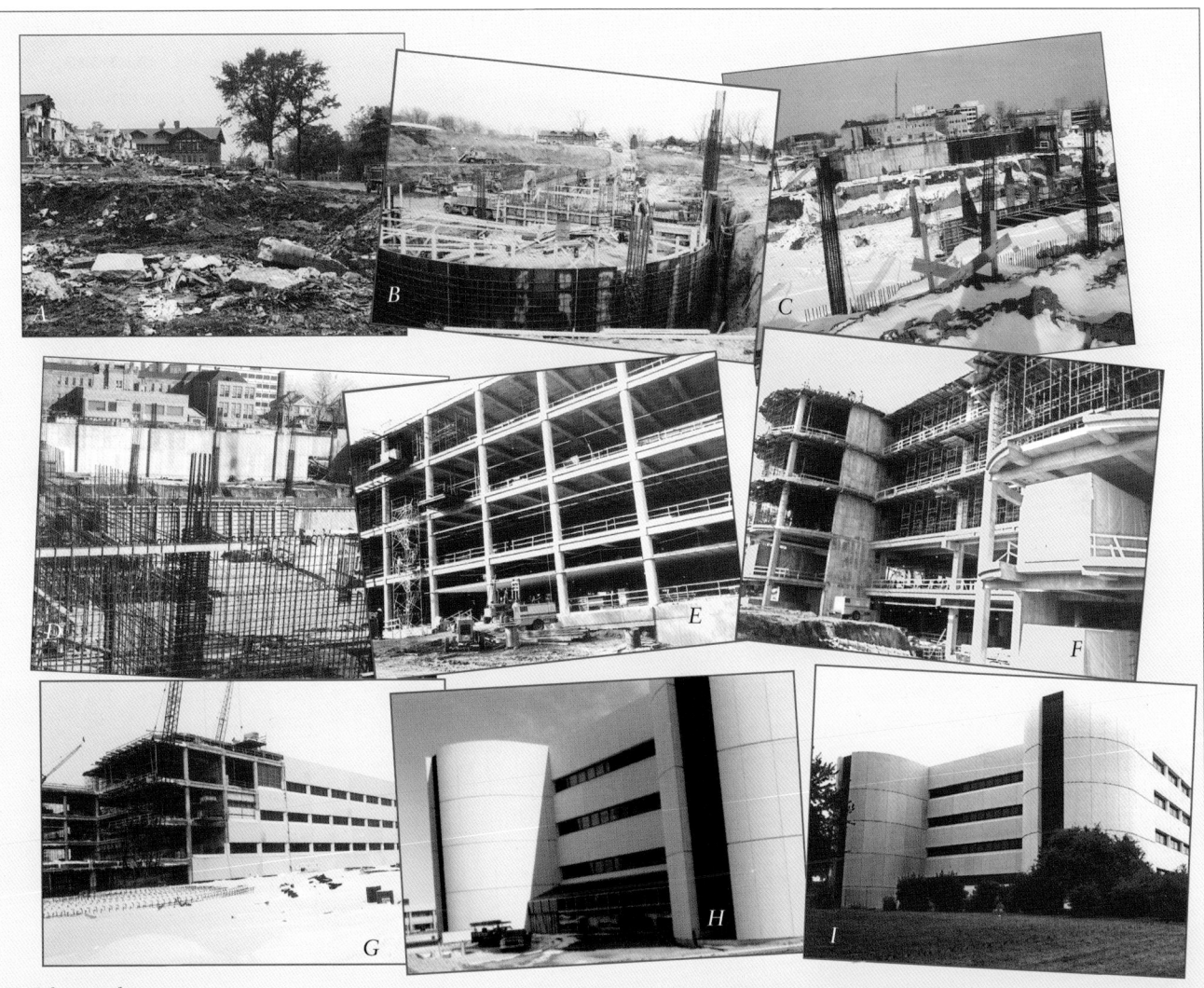

A hospital emerges —

A One week after the official groundbreaking ceremonies in September 1977, old County buildings were razed and construction had officially begun.
B By the middle of November, the excavation was complete and footings were being poured.
C A cold and snowy January 1978 revealed progress on the hospital.
D As spring began, more of the hospital was evident to onlookers.
E August revealed additional details of the framing and mechanicals.
F In September, the distinctive architecture of Froedtert Hospital became more visible.
G By January 1979, the promise of Froedtert became apparent.
H In March 1980, the West Entrance was nearly ready to welcome patients and visitors.
I With summer came the landscaping at the east end of the hospital.

changing interior walls to accommodate new services or technology. Even in its original design, Froedtert was committed to the same philosophy that it holds today of logical, not lavish, construction.

At Roe's suggestion, the Building Committee agreed to undertake the construction on a "fast track" system where bids could go out as plans were completed. This method would save time and money and provide the flexibility needed to meet engineering and technology changes during the three-year construction timetable for the hospital.

"The typical way to build is to go right down to the final working drawings and send these out for bid," Roe said. "By going with the preliminary drawings, we saved a year to a year-and-a-half of construction time as well as substantial sums of money." There are risks in an undertaking of this sort, however. Gerd Zoller was the construction manager for the Madison firm of Findorff–Hutter, the hospital's general contractor. Based on the preliminary drawings, Zoller guaranteed a construction cost of $39 million. As final drawings were completed and bids were returned from subcontractors, Findorff discovered that the guaranteed price was $2 million short of the total cost. Faced with this bad news, Findorff argued that the architects had designed high-cost items in the detailed drawings. At first, the architects were reluctant to change any aspect of the design details. Eventually through compromise, some costs and risks were reduced. However, when the building was completed, the two parties ended up settling their financial differences in court. ■

Chapter 23

Merger Problems

As construction of Froedtert Hospital progressed, the mandated hospital merger reached an impasse. The mergers were an integral part of the state's approval for Froedtert. Negotiations began in mid-1977 and escalated into one of the most confusing and complex events in the history of Milwaukee hospitals. When the three hospitals continued to struggle over the details of a merger, the area health planning agency invoked its mandatory arbitration clause that was included in the Froedtert approval. Walter McNerney, president of the national Blue Cross Association, was retained by the health planning agency as an arbitrator. McNerney completed his negotiations in late November 1977, recommending that Lutheran and Deaconess merge, while Froedtert could be added later. Annual savings of $12 million to $18 million would result from merged Deaconess and Lutheran operations. Both hospitals approved McNerney's recommendations.

The major stumbling block centered on management of the merged hospital corporation. Three months passed, and the merger was nowhere near completion. Then in February 1978, Lutheran officials proposed a management plan that placed Roe as president and CEO of the new hospital corporation with Ken Jamron, president of Deaconess, serving as chief operating officer. At this point, Roe was also president of Froedtert. Deaconess officials rejected the Lutheran plan and countered with one of their own. Ken Jamron should be the CEO of the merged hospital corporation. Dean Roe should not be an employee of the new corporation but be retained as a consultant during the transition period. This plan was rejected by Lutheran officials. By the end of February, Deaconess announced its withdrawal from any further merger talks with Lutheran Hospital and, in a parting statement, said that the withdrawal also applied to any negotiations involving Froedtert Hospital.

In early June 1978, the Medical College began its move from the Marquette University campus to its new home at the medical center. The school also contracted with the Burroughs Corporation to form a Joint Medical Computer Services Center.

Mainframe hardware would be located at the Medical College. Froedtert and Lutheran hospitals signed on to access Burroughs' state-of-the-art patient care and financial software programs. The idea behind the formation of the Service Center was development of an income source by selling the patient care and financial software to other hospitals. Froedtert's construction continued on schedule despite the fact that a Deaconess-Lutheran merger was in limbo. The elements of an academic medical center were falling into place—or so it seemed. ■

Chapter 24

Problems at County General Hospital

In 1978, concerns were beginning to be raised about County General Hospital and its role as a key element in the developing medical center. Two major problems affected County General's patient volume. Medicare and Medicaid patients could now choose any hospital for care. Emergency cases that previously were conveyed to County General were now being admitted to any hospital, further decreasing patient volume. The hospital's daily charge—highest in the area—made it difficult to compete for the private-pay patients. The higher costs at County General were attributed to its support of medical education and its share of costs to support the Milwaukee County Courthouse departments for legal work, personnel, data processing, interest payments, and maintenance of vacant or unassigned portions of County buildings. These cross charges added to the daily patient service costs while the decrease in patient volume seriously affected the financial stability of the hospital.

In view of these circumstances, officials raised questions about the hospital's future ability to provide care and patient access to its services. The situation at the County Hospital was reaching a critical state. Over the years, the problems were voiced by elected County officials as well as by hospital administration.

Early in 1978, the County Board retained Hyatt and Associates, a management consulting firm, to study the hospital's operations. A preliminary report by the Hyatt group indicated a probable change in the role of the hospital. This suggestion brought a surprising response from Supervisor Emil Stanislawski, chair of the County Board Finance Committee. Stanislawski indicated that the County Board might be looking to lease or sell the hospital to the Medical College of Wisconsin as a means of property tax relief. He felt that the role of the County in healthcare needed to be re-evaluated. Some supervisors questioned whether the County should continue to provide services to the indigent sick or purchase the care from other hospitals.

Symuel Smith, appointed director of County Institutions in spring 1978, stated that the system of controls on the hospital's administration should be changed.

He said the hospital reported to too many County committees and boards. He acknowledged that the County Board should set policy and program services, but hospital administrators should be responsible for day-to-day management. The observations were made at a time when County Hospital's operating deficit for 1978 was projected at $5 million. The hospital's deficit in 1977 was $4.9 million. Some suggested that the hospital be sold to the state or that the state should pay for care of the indigent sick.

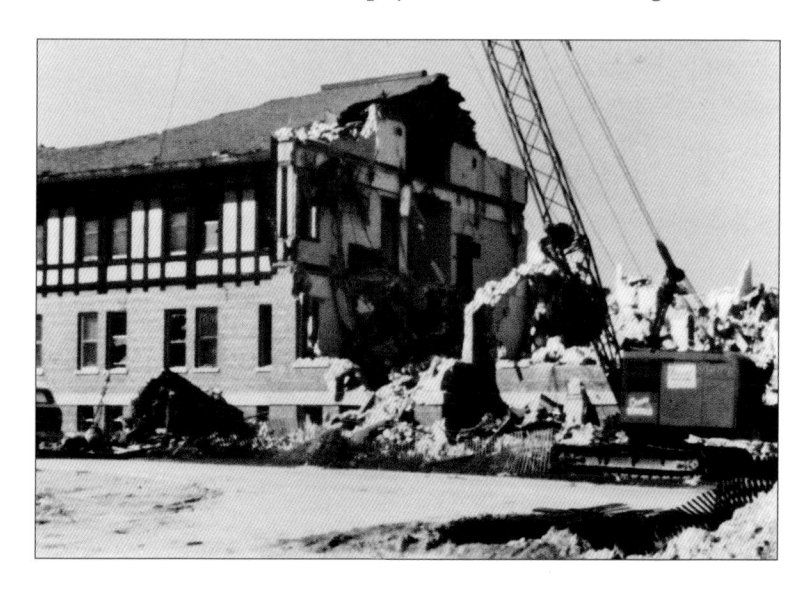

Making room on the County Institutions Grounds for Froedtert Hospital

Even though the County Board had retained the Hyatt consulting firm, County Executive O'Donnell appointed David Carley, former Medical College president, to study the future role of the hospital. O'Donnell felt that Carley's experience in health and medical issues would bring about a sound analysis of County Hospital's problems. Not to be upstaged in this flurry of studies, the County Board undertook its own review of the problem. Supervisor James Krivitz headed a team that included representatives from government, labor, private hospitals, the Medical College, the planning agency, and the Citizen's Governmental Research Bureau. In 1978, there were three separate studies underway seeking solutions to County General's problems.

By late spring and early summer 1979, preliminary findings and recommendations were unveiled from these studies. Carley's report called for major administrative and management changes at County General, including a new governing structure for the County's health facilities. The Hyatt consultant's report recommended a board to have nearly complete authority over operations of County General Hospital and the Mental Health Center. The study by County Supervisor James Krivitz's committee echoed that suggestion. All three studies agreed that budget and policy determinations be left to the County Board with a separate body to assume responsibility for hospital operations.

In early fall 1979, County Executive William O'Donnell proposed a complete reorganization of the medical center. In a *Milwaukee Journal* story of October 7, 1979, O'Donnell was quoted as saying, "We pretend our status is that of a geographic member of the medical center while in reality, we choose to maintain our firm position as landlord, lawgiver and big-brother guardian. The greatest transgression is perpetuated by Milwaukee County itself."

O'Donnell proposed creation of a Milwaukee County Services Board of community members, headed by the chair of the County Board's Health Committee; it would operate under the Board of Supervisors. However, administrative direction would be removed from County Board committees. It was the County Board's committee structure that often delayed decisions affecting hospital operation. The plan would empower the executive committee of the Services Board to set rates for services, invest surplus funds, employ staff, and contract for goods and services to carry out its duties. O'Donnell said this board could take over from Milwaukee County the job of pushing through the shared services facility—the Bridge Building. The proposed Services Board would sponsor the facility and charge fees to the institutions that used it. O'Donnell's plan included some of the recommended changes made in the other studies. His plan would require a change in state legislation. While there was merit to these recommendations, not one was implemented. The status quo remained.

Instead of a $41 million facility housing emergency services, laboratories, radiology, surgery, and clinics, a more modest structure was proposed. The revised plan called for an insulated and heated two-level corridor between Froedtert and County hospitals. This structure would enable movement of patients and staff between the two hospitals and serve as the base for future construction of a shared service facility. There was doubt that approval and construction of the corridor could be completed by the time Froedtert opened in mid-1980. Without some connecting structure, Froedtert would be isolated from County General. That proved to be the case when Froedtert opened in 1980. There was nothing but five hundred feet of open space between the two hospitals. In fact, the Bridge Building did not open until 1988. ∎

Chapter 25

Building a Hospital and a Staff

Dean Roe moved to Froedtert's temporary headquarters in an office building at Bluemound and Mayfair roads. Margaret Fuchs, who had worked with him for many years, comprised his entire staff. Soon after, Joyce Brunau moved from her duties as executive administrative assistant at Lutheran to a similar role at Froedtert. Brunau remains in that position at Froedtert and at the time of this writing is the longest tenured hospital staff member. She has been privy to all of the interesting facets of Froedtert's struggle for approval, and she has witnessed the political intrigue surrounding the hospital's history and development of the medical center. Brunau has been the integral link between the administrations of Dean Roe and William Petasnick, serving as an invaluable resource to this correspondent and the administrative team as well. Above all, integrity has consistently remained the hallmark of her personal and professional life

Roe welcomed the opportunity to completely organize a new hospital:

Getting Froedtert ready was an opportunity of a professional lifetime. I was literally given a blank sheet of paper. There was nobody there at Froedtert when I began as the chief executive officer. I could start with what the hospital was going to be like, the people I would hire, the policies we were going to have, the directions we were going to take. It was a dream opportunity for someone in the hospital field, and an opportunity that few hospital executives get to experience. It's similar to a blank canvas facing an artist. You have the opportunity to create an organization defined to fulfill the mission of healthcare, education, and research.

However, at the close of 1979, another red flag was raised by the local health planning agency when it questioned Froedtert's order for a $700,000 CAT scanner. Litigation seemed to be the only alternative route to a resolution. The controversy would extend for months as Froedtert began assembling its medical and hospital staff for an early summer opening in 1980.

Other problems of greater magnitude included more litigation over a final construction cost overrun, a sizeable outlay for its share of construction costs for the two-level connector planned between the two hospitals, and legal and penalty costs involved in the hospital information systems contract among Froedtert and Lutheran hospitals and the Medical College. Resolution of these problems involved litigation and non-budgeted expenses that directly affected the viability of Froedtert Hospital in its first years of operation. These were busy days for Wayne Roper, who successfully represented Froedtert's interests in all the litigation.

In the CAT scanner controversy, Froedtert officials said that the intent to purchase the scanner was included in the hospital construction plan approved by the state in 1977. Health planners said that references to the scanner in the construction application were not direct enough and agency approval was needed. The controversy arose shortly after the planning agency completed a study of area hospitals and scanner services. Six hospitals were listed as suitable sites for scanners based on quality, cost, accessibility, and availability. Froedtert was not listed because it was felt that the hospital could share the two scanners at County General and avoid duplication.

Dean Roe, Froedtert's First Chief Executive Officer

The adage fits Dean K. Roe: He was the right man at the right time and place in Froedtert's history.

Roe served twenty-three years as the first president/CEO of Froedtert Hospital, from 1970 until his retirement in 1993. His undergraduate degree was earned at St. Olaf College and his master's degree in healthcare administration from the University of Minnesota.

Prior to his career at Froedtert, his professional experience included nine years as assistant administrator at Northwestern and Fairview hospitals in Minneapolis. Roe came to Milwaukee "on loan" from the Fairview Hospital administration to serve as executive director of Milwaukee Psychiatric Hospital in Wauwatosa. That was at the request of James A. Hamilton and Associates, the Minneapolis consulting firm that needed on-site assistance for a management study that Hamilton was conducting for the psychiatric facility.

While he was executive director of the psychiatric hospital, Roe was retained by the Froedtert trustees as a consultant in their planning efforts for Froedtert Hospital. His role and relationship to Froedtert Hospital as president and as a consultant to the trustees covers a thirty-one-year span. In those years, he displayed a quiet but consistent leadership role in defining and maintaining the position of Froedtert as a vital resource for patient care, clinical research, and education in an academic medical setting. He was known for his deliberate study of problems and opportunities, and for his decisiveness in implementing change to strengthen the mission and purpose of Froedtert Hospital.

Roe served as president of the Wisconsin State Hospital Association and the Milwaukee Hospital Council. He also served on the Wisconsin Health and Education Authority for twelve years and on the Wisconsin Rate Review Committee. He was a member of several key committees of the American Hospital Association and a board member of Blue Cross, the Milwaukee Regional Medical Center, and Froedtert Hospital.

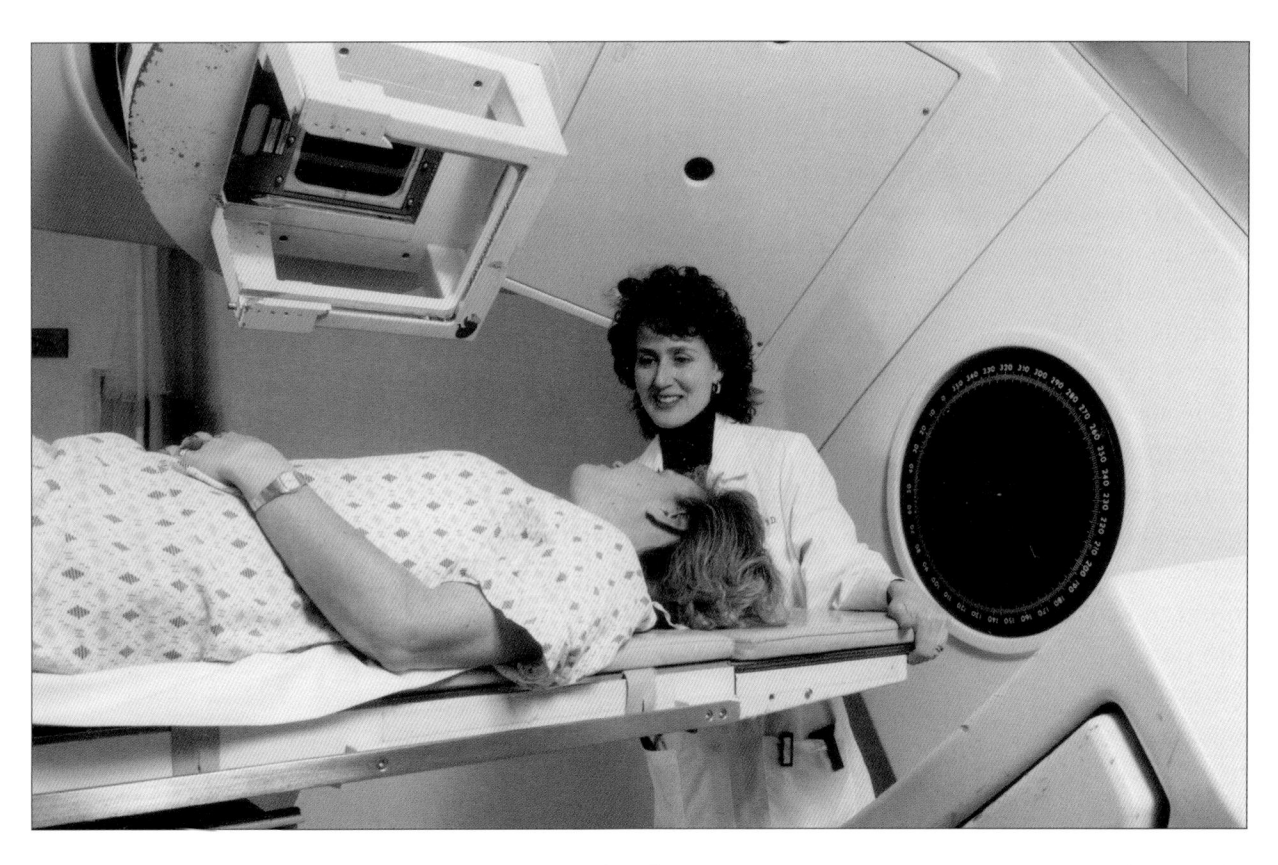

A CAT scanner such as this one was the source of controversy as Froedtert believed that its purchase had been approved in the original proposal, while health planning officials said it was not approved.

Convinced that state approval for the scanner had been granted in the original construction application, Froedtert filed a lawsuit naming the State Department of Health and Social Services as defendants. After months of litigation, the court ruled in Froedtert's favor. But the decision was not rendered until after Froedtert had opened its doors in the fall of 1980 without a scanner in place. With no diagnostic scanners and five hundred feet of open space between the two hospitals, Froedtert patients had to be transported by private ambulance to County Hospital for CAT scans. The costs of transporting patients for CAT scans at County were borne by Froedtert. The daily volume of CAT patient transports were often as high as fifteen.

While the scanner problem was in litigation, state planners created more controversy for Froedtert and County hospitals. Before it would approve the application for the two-level connector, the state demanded a long-range plan involving Froedtert, County General, and the Medical College. County officials found additional requests by state officials for additional information unacceptable. A dispute on the county-state agreement further delayed an approval for the corridor link.

More problems arose when County General nurses, in a war over wages, began an exodus to other hospitals. The nurses' departures forced some patient units to close, causing substantial revenue losses. County Supervisor Daniel Casey called for County General to merge with Froedtert as a private institution to cut property taxes and increase efficiency.

Meanwhile Froedtert's picture was colored with a predicted cost overrun on construction and the possibility that the heating and air conditioning system would be extremely expensive to operate. The California architects had not taken into consideration Milwaukee's humid summers and frigid winters. The system had a 100 percent exchange of air. All internal heated or conditioned air was not recirculated but continuously replaced. The high cost of this system had a direct and costly effect on the hospital's financial status in its early years of operation. Eventually a retrofit of the entire system was necessary.

In the spring and summer months of 1980, building and trade unions were in negotiations for new contracts. The likelihood of prolonged strikes by a number of trades seemed inevitable. Froedtert's construction was in its final stages when the carpenters union went on strike the first week in June. It marked the first time that the carpenters had walked off job sites in more than a decade. Much of the finish work, including drywall for patient rooms and common areas, came to a standstill. A summer opening of the hospital was out of the question. Despite the delay, Froedtert's administrative staff continued working on the organization of resources for the opening day, now projected for late summer or early fall. ■

Part Four

1980-2005

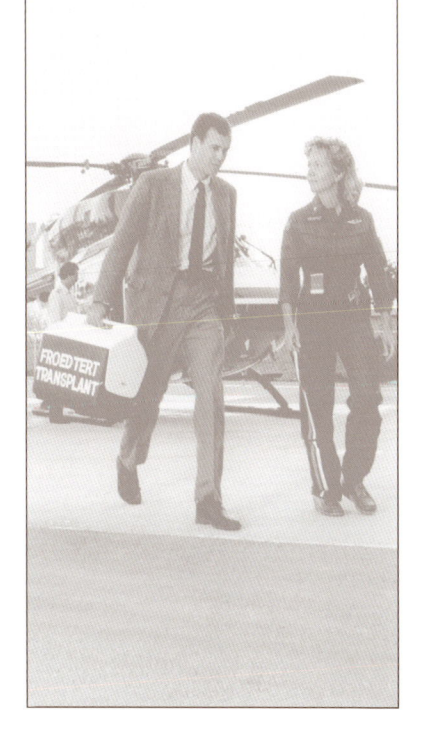

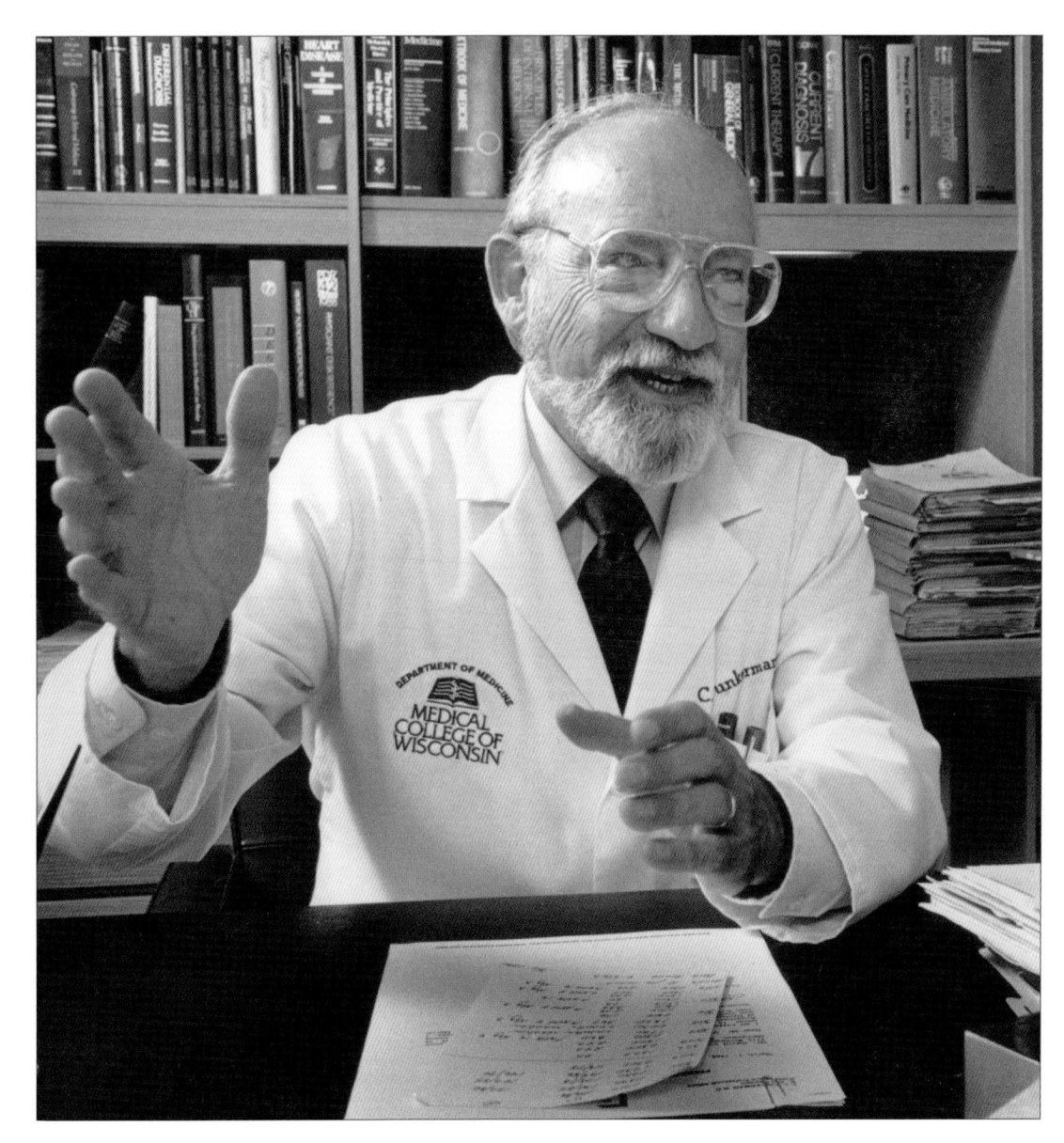

Dr. Carl Junkerman had responsibility for organizing the medical staffs for Froedtert and County General hospitals.

Chapter 26

Organizing the Staff

In the intense competition for nurses in the Milwaukee area, Froedtert's nursing administration introduced a scheduling system that would give the new hospital a competitive edge in recruiting staff. Mary Larter, vice president of Patient Services, had devised the scheduling system for Evergreen Hospital in Seattle. The staffing plan called for nurses to work ten-hour shifts for seven days, followed by a full week off when an alternate team assumed patient care service. Called the 7-70 plan, it was the first of its kind in the Midwest and proved to be a highly effective nurse recruitment tool for Froedtert.

Larter's system gave nurses the opportunity to schedule their professional and private lives a whole year in advance. She believed that existing systems created havoc with nurses' lives. The 7-70 plan eliminated irregular hours, shift rotations, split days off, and infrequent weekends off. A nurse earning a week's vacation in the first year of employment would have three weeks off. The one-week vacation period fell between the weeks when the nurse was off duty under the 7-70 system.

There were other advantages to the 7-70 system as well.

A key factor in patient satisfaction is the quality of nursing care. Accordingly, a decentralized system of patient care was adopted at Froedtert and it is still in place today. Nurses set policies and procedures as they apply to the needs of surgical patients in one unit or medical patients in another. The nurse-to-patient ratio is high in this system.

The system benefits both patients and nursing personnel. Because shifts overlap, the ratio of nurses to patients is higher at peak periods, creating more direct registered nurse care for routine as well as special patient needs. Overlapping shifts reduces fatigue and allows nurses to have more frequent communication and contact with patients and family members. The program is so innovative that it won a Milwaukee *Small Business Times* Health Care Hero Award for corporate achievement in 2005.

At the outset, Dr. Carl Junkerman, senior vice president for Professional and Academic Affairs, organized the medical staff. A special committee of faculty members, including Dr. Jerry DeCosse, then chairman of Surgery, and Dr. Daniel McCarty, then chairman of Medicine, decided which services would be moved from County to Froedtert. After long deliberations on the location of services at Froedtert and County hospitals, the faculty committee turned the decision over to administration.

Roe recalled the final outcome on the decisions surrounding the location of services:

> We made some decisions rather arbitrarily but with economic and clinical relationships in mind. For instance, we would not separate services such as Neurology from Neurosurgery. Eventually we settled on the fourteen services that would move to Froedtert. There were a lot of program directors who did not want to come here and some who wanted to come to Froedtert but did not.

The services moved to Froedtert included Anesthesiology, Dermatology, Endocrine Metabolic, Gastroenterology, Neurology, Neurosurgery, Nephrology, Oral Surgery, Otolaryngology, Pulmonary Medicine, Plastic and Reconstructive Surgery, and Urology. Not all services were in place at Froedtert when it opened. Some were delayed a few months for a variety of reasons.

A unique agreement was reached on the operation and billing of radiology and laboratory services for the two hospitals. Radiology services would be sold to County General by Froedtert. County General would sell laboratory services to Froedtert. This agreement caused delays in payments for services from both sides of the table. Eventually the inequities of service and billing between these two diagnostic services would result in formation of United Regional Medical Services, an independent service organization contracting with both hospitals to provide services more efficiently and equitably.

To insure an adequate caseload for care and teaching purposes, the two hospitals alternated medical emergency admissions. In one twenty-four-hour period, all medical emergency cases would be hospitalized at County General. In the next twenty-four hours, the medical emergencies would be admitted to Froedtert. Emergency and trauma cases requiring specialty care were referred to the hospital providing that service. Patients with severe head trauma went to Froedtert's neuroscience service while cardiac cases stayed at County General.

All outpatient services were to be provided in the clinics at County Hospital, including the fourteen specialties located at Froedtert. Ultimately this proved to be a rather untenable situation for the medical staff at Froedtert. Without a connecting corridor between the hospitals, Froedtert physicians walked through all types of weather to staff outpatient clinics at County. Some of the

Froedtert specialties began establishing outpatient services using inpatient rooms that had not been opened for service at Froedtert before eventually moving into the West and East Clinics.

By April 1980, managers for twenty-one departments or services at Froedtert began establishing policies and procedures. The summer months of organizing the new hospital were chaotic, confusing, frustrating, humorous, and unifying. Staff members who endured that tumultuous summer fondly recall the spirit of cooperation between clinical and administrative staff as the major factor that enabled the hospital to be ready for its first patients.

Because many areas of the hospital were unfinished, work space was limited in the six months prior to opening. The administrative staff worked in a large open area eventually occupied by the hospital's Family Center. Nursing staff and other clinical departments worked across the courtyard. There were no cubicles or interior walls separating work space for department heads and directors. Desks were aligned just inches apart. Files were kept in cardboard boxes, since whole departments would be forced to move frequently when construction crews moved in for finish work and to set up cubicles. Work days of ten to twelve hours were the norm.

Recruiting staff through those months had some rather peculiar twists. Prospective staff members had to wear hard hats during interviews. Recruiting tours meant climbing over rolls of carpeting and avoiding wires hanging from the ceilings. Pizza parties became part of the recruitment process, since the hospital's dietary department was not completed. Local vendors enjoyed boom times delivering pizzas to the hospital on a daily basis.

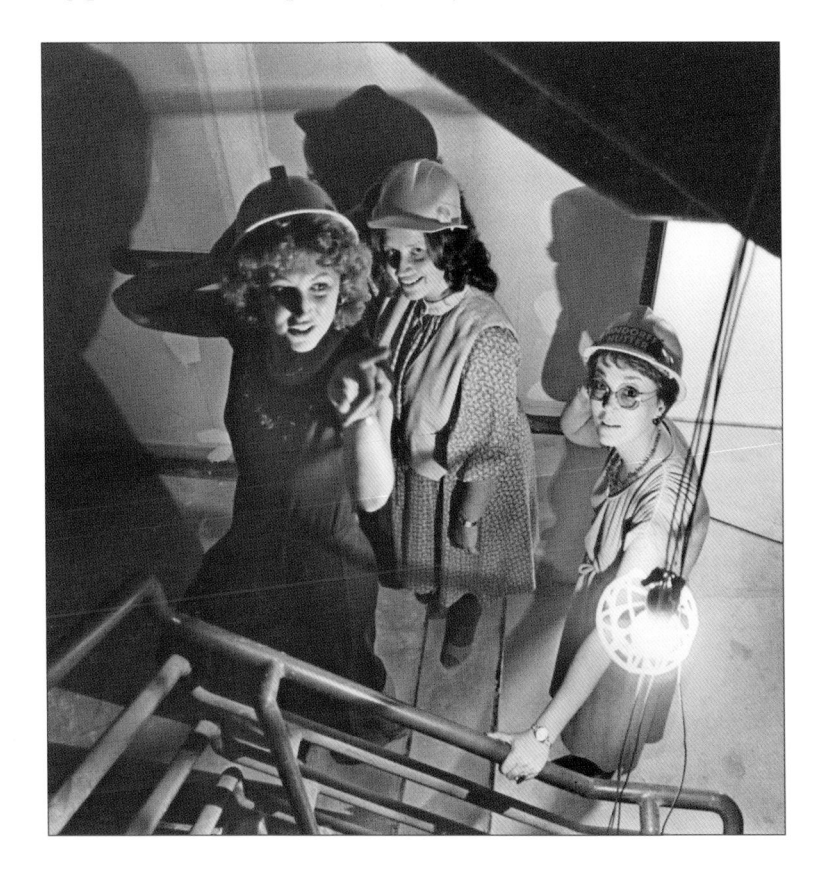

Among the applicants for staff and middle management positions during that summer was a middle school teacher who applied for a supervisory position in the plant operations department. Eventually

Left to right: Staff members Pat Profit, Jackie (Schaeffer) Davis, and Sue Senelly

that former middle school science and mathematics teacher, John Balzer, became vice president for Facility Planning and Development. Since then, Balzer has been responsible for planning and overseeing construction and renovations projects at Froedtert valued at more than $100 million. Other early staffers include Pam Maxson-Cooper, who began as a staff nurse in the neurosurgery patient unit and moved through the ranks to become senior vice president for Patient Care Services and chief nursing officer, overseeing a staff of more than fifteen hundred nursing personnel. While not on the staff when the hospital opened, Cathy Buck became a staff nurse a few months later. Her clinical skills in patient care soon moved her to director of Patient Care and then to director of Outpatient Dialysis. She rose to the position of executive vice president and chief operating officer. These are just three examples of the many talented staff members whose commitment and leadership assured Froedtert's long-standing reputation of excellence.

Chapter 27

Opening Day!

Opening day! The formal dedication was September 29, 1980. Governor Lee Dreyfus was the principal speaker. Preceding the dedication ceremonies, the Froedtert Board of Directors hosted a special tour for Mary Froedtert and her children and grandchildren. More than six hundred people gathered in the West Hospital courtyard to hear the Wisconsin governor deliver the dedication speech. While the chief executive spoke, the first admission to Froedtert took place. A Fond du Lac man with a heart problem was admitted to Froedtert and then transferred to County Hospital's cardiology service. Three other patients were admitted that afternoon. It was a small beginning and a dream fulfilled.

By the end of that memorable opening day, another significant event took place. Lutheran and Deaconess hospitals signed a merger agreement. Children's Hospital continued to express interest in constructing its new hospital on the Lutheran Hospital site at North 22nd Street and West Kilbourn Avenue.

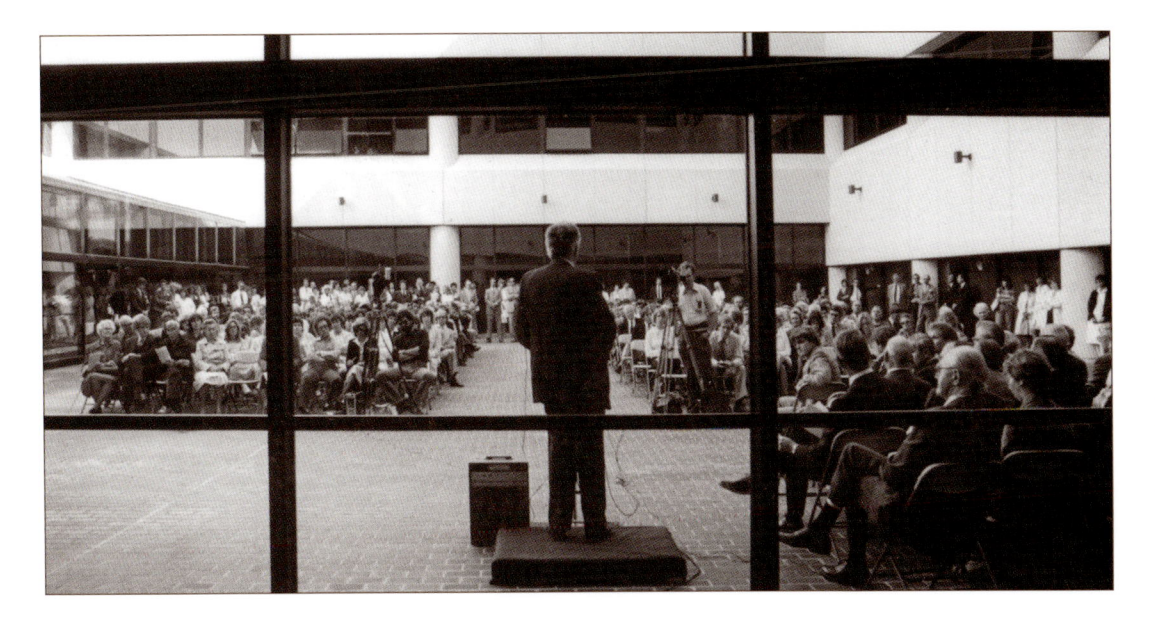

It was "standing room only" at the dedication ceremonies. Governor Lee Sherman Dreyfus was the keynote speaker.

Wauwatosans for Tomorrow Become Froedtert's First Volunteers

As the summer of 1980 heated up, so did preparations for the opening of Froedtert Hospital. Amid all the activity, it became clear that the new hospital was going to need help—before it even opened.

There was no auxiliary or volunteer service group organized at Froedtert, but there was a need for extra hands during the public open house tours. The solution to this problem came in a roundabout way. The hospital received a midsummer call from Alice Krebs, representing a civic organization known as the Wauwatosans for Tomorrow. The group wanted an early tour of the new hospital. In the interest of fostering a strong relationship with the Wauwatosa community, the hospital happily agreed to host a tour and reception. In late July, more than forty Wauwatosa citizens took the tour and enjoyed a wine and cheese reception in the fourth-floor courtyard. No one realized the importance of this community event that night.

As the hospital opening drew near, the problem of staffing the public tours remained. A call went out to Mrs. Krebs for help from her civic group. When told that at least fifty volunteers would be needed, she replied, "You've got them." She and Mary Wilkinson, a Wauwatosa Common Council member, recruited more than fifty Wauwatosans for Tomorrow members to help with the public tours. They were vital in handing out information and guiding the more than eight thousand people touring Froedtert on that beautiful weekend of September 12 and 13, 1980.

Alice Krebs' organizational skills and community contacts did not go unnoticed by the Froedtert Administration. She was their choice to organize an auxiliary at Froedtert. Many of the Wauwatosans for Tomorrow became founding members of the Froedtert Hospital Auxiliary. Under her direction for the next ten years, the Auxiliary donated thousands of service hours to the hospital and nearly $1 million in support of numerous hospital projects and programs.

Before the hospital marked its first anniversary, volunteers numbered eighty-five. They had established a gift shop where many worked. Some were patient escorts, while still others worked at the information desk or delivered menus, mail, and flowers to patients. Three years later, their ranks had reached 150 who helped in pharmacy, dietary, several clinics, materials processing and distribution, patient transportation, and admitting, as well as the gift shop. Today few, if any, departments at Froedtert are not served by volunteers.

The first major undertaking for the volunteer group was the landscaping of the courtyard just inside the original front entrance to the hospital. The raised flower beds and graceful trees brought a welcome and warm change to the precast concrete and brick surroundings in 1983. The more than $1.5 million in gifts to the hospital that volunteers have contributed over the years have ranged from the dramatic to the mundane. Examples of their many contributions include new medical equipment, copy machines, a player piano, and landscaping for the North Tower Courtyard.

When Froedtert marked its twenty-five years of service to the community, five Froedtert volunteers were also recognized for their twenty-five years of service to the hospital: Pauline Fichtner, Bernice and Bob Henderson, Mary Alice Smith, and Maggie Von Kohn.

Then Auxiliary President Carla Hering presented a check for $45,000 to Froedtert Board President Thomas Smallwood (left) and Froedtert President and CEO William Petasnick in 1998. Over the years, the Auxiliary, now the Volunteer Associates, has contributed more than $1.5 million to Froedtert Hospital.

Chapter 28

The Changing Hospital Scene

While the patient census remained modest at Froedtert, the demand for beds in the metropolitan area increased dramatically. Elective medical and surgical admissions were being delayed due to a shortage of available beds, and some hospitals stopped accepting emergency admissions.

Within weeks of Froedtert's opening, local hospitals filed letters of intent to add beds or renovate services in the amount of $150 million. The proposals were surprising in view of the planning agency's position that there were excess beds in the area. The cost of these proposed expansions drew the interest of the Greater Milwaukee Committee and the Metropolitan Milwaukee Association of Commerce. The two organizations formed a task force to examine methods of containing and controlling the costs of healthcare. The leadership of both groups envisioned a system where there would be fewer hospitals in the area. To determine what changes would be needed in healthcare services, the two associations asked the health planning agency to develop a short-range plan with an eye toward a master plan.

The Southeastern Wisconsin Health Systems Agency (SEWHSA) established the Interim Guidance Committee to devise a plan to contain duplication of services and excess beds. By the end of 1980, the Interim Guidance Committee drafted three plans to organize a hospital system. In January 1981, the interim plans received extensive media coverage. Under the plans, as many as eight hospitals in the Milwaukee area would be closed. Of special concern was a recommendation that Children's Hospital be incorporated in a seventy-five-bed tertiary care unit at the Milwaukee Regional Medical Center. A thirty-bed pediatric primary care and walk-in service would be located at Mount Sinai. One alternative called for closing pediatric services at three community hospitals and reducing beds in others. Another had Lutheran, Deaconess, and Milwaukee Psychiatric hospitals located at a single site. As it was, Deaconess and Lutheran officials had already agreed to consolidate all services on the Lutheran site. The two consolidated hospitals would be renamed the Good Samaritan Medical Center.

All three plans suggested closures of services in heart surgery, CAT scanning, and radiation therapy at designated hospitals. The alternative plans to close hospitals brought adverse reactions to Froedtert Hospital's existence. Questions were raised as to why the new Froedtert Hospital was operating when old-line hospitals were being asked to close. The plans represented a carload of fireworks awaiting ignition. Reaction was swift.

The proposed plans created a firestorm of response at public hearings scheduled throughout the seven-county health planning area. In Waukesha, overflow crowds created a health and safety issue, forcing an early closing of the public hearing. Hospitals initiated advertising campaigns and communication programs to plead their respective cases. The hospitals designated for closure under the plan sent busloads of personnel to the public hearings. They carried hand-painted signs critical of the plan and urging support of their respective hospitals. City of Milwaukee officials decried the plan to close six downtown hospitals.

The Medical Society of Milwaukee County also weighed in on the issue. It suggested closing County General, St. Anthony, and Foundation hospitals, stating that Froedtert now represented an excellent on-site teaching hospital for the Medical College and recommended that County's services be consolidated at Froedtert. The Society's report recommended that Children's Hospital be maintained as an independent, two-hundred-bed regional pediatric center.

The adverse public reaction to the interim plans was loud and clear, and SEWHSA shelved the plans. For the second time in three years, a plan for downtown medical services was rejected by health officials and the general public. New efforts were then scheduled to design a health plan for the 1980s whereby planning would be carried out by representative study groups to insure that all sides were represented in planning efforts. The study groups faced a possible time deadline. At this time, the federal government was debating the issue of continuing to suspend or reduce support for regional planning agencies. ■

Chapter 29

Troublesome Times Ahead

Unforeseen financial problems created a critical period in the first years of Froedtert's operation. Shifting existing referral patterns from long-established medical centers outside of Southeastern Wisconsin proved to be more difficult than anticipated. In its first year of operation, fewer than two thousand referrals were made to Froedtert. Private practice physicians holding medical school clinical faculty appointments were granted privileges to admit patients and teach at Froedtert, but these community physicians soon found it difficult to juggle patient admissions to more than one hospital and still fulfill their teaching responsibilities at Froedtert. The attrition of these community physicians affected the inpatient census at a time when Froedtert needed patient volume.

Financial obligations further drained the operating budget. Froedtert agreed to pay $1.7 million as its share of the construction costs for the connecting tunnel to Milwaukee County Hospital. Also, since Samaritan Hospital had never used the new Burroughs computer system, the court absolved Samaritan from its financial obligations for the new system. As a result, the costs would be divided two, not three, ways. Froedtert and the Medical College had to divide the initial costs as well as the monthly service costs of the Burroughs system between themselves.

By mid-1982 and into 1983, inpatient volume fell short of budget projections. In its first three years, Froedtert suffered operating losses of nearly $9 million. To trim more than $1 million from the operating budget, staff hours were reduced in some departments, as were wages and salaries. A freeze on hiring was instituted, and there were two moderate layoffs of middle management and other hospital staff. To keep the hospital operation viable, the Froedtert Trust provided funding to offset some of the financial losses.

Other factors contributed to Froedtert's early difficulties. Occupancy rates for all hospitals throughout Southeastern Wisconsin fell substantially during this period, with some reporting volumes as low as 65 percent. These inpatient declines in the Milwaukee area followed a nationwide pattern: an economic downturn and layoffs increased the number of people without health insurance.

The federal government added to the nation's hospital woes by establishing Diagnosis Related Groups (DRGs) in 1984. Hospitals were reimbursed according to a fixed schedule of payments for 467 diagnostic and therapeutic procedures. The plan was a major revision of the Medicare reimbursement formula. Previously Medicare paid hospitals and physicians for reasonable costs of service. Under the new plan, if costs exceeded the set fee for a particular test or treatment, hospitals would then absorb the loss. When service costs were less than the fixed fee, hospitals could keep the difference. To accommodate a portion of medical education costs, teaching hospitals received an additional 5 percent over the fixed DRG fee. But within three years this percentage was reduced.

County General Hospital also began to experience reduced inpatient volume, with predictions of substantial financial losses. In the mid-1980s, County Institutions officials formed a committee to explore the possibilities of selling or leasing the hospital or turning it over to a private firm. At this stage, no action was taken, but the concept of a major change in the County Hospital mission and purpose would be visited again in future years.

Conversely, while hospitals' inpatient volumes were declining, the demand for outpatient care was growing substantially. The competition for outpatient revenue in Milwaukee was fierce. In the scramble to claim a share of this new market, a rash of outpatient clinics and urgent care centers opened in the Milwaukee metro area. Despite their hospital affiliations, physicians formed competing outpatient services within their office settings or in vacated retail stores, filling stations, and restaurants. One Milwaukee physician group remodeled a filling station, while another took over a hamburger stand as an urgent care and outpatient clinic. With their higher operating costs, hospitals couldn't compete with these freestanding outpatient and urgent care clinics. Dean Roe developed a plan that called for the establishment of affiliates that could be utilized as centers to generate revenue for Froedtert.

As a limited partner, the Froedtert Trust invested in an outpatient clinic with the Milwaukee Medical Clinic on the southwest side to develop an inpatient referral source for Froedtert and capture some of the outpatient revenue. The clinic did not meet expectations and was eventually closed, as were many others.

Despite the tenuous financial condition of Froedtert in these early years, the hospital had to weigh financial risks in acquiring state-of-the-art technology against long-term benefits for the hospital and the publics it served. The hospital had to establish itself as an accessible referral source for complex medical and surgical cases. As referrals increased, its tertiary mission for referrals began to gain statewide recognition.

Medical College physicians and hospital staff introduced new procedures and technology not previously available to residents of Southeastern Wisconsin. The plan was to highlight these services through the media and have Froedtert medical staff conduct teaching seminars for community physicians on campus and in community hospitals. A number of accomplishments attracted media and referring physicians' attention in these formative years. They included limb replants and free flap surgeries; a unique affiliation with GE Medical Systems; discoveries made in the Clinical Research Laboratory; and the burgeoning organ transplant program.

Froedtert established itself as the preeminent center for replanting severed hands, arms, legs, and other extremities, becoming one of the largest such centers in the country. The microvascular skills of the plastic surgery team of Drs. Hani Matloub, John Yousif, and James Sanger gained worldwide attention in a very unusual case. An industrial accident resulted in amputations of finger tips, fingers, and a hand of a young man. In a procedure that lasted more than twenty-nine hours, the surgeons reattached the tips to four fingers, then reattached the fingers to the severed hand, and then reattached the hand to the arm. At the time, it was the only three-level limb replant successfully completed anywhere in the world.

This photo from the 1980s shows a patient receiving physical therapy at the Hand Center. Today Froedtert & the Medical College of Wisconsin Hand Center provides exceptional treatment for all parts of the upper extremities.

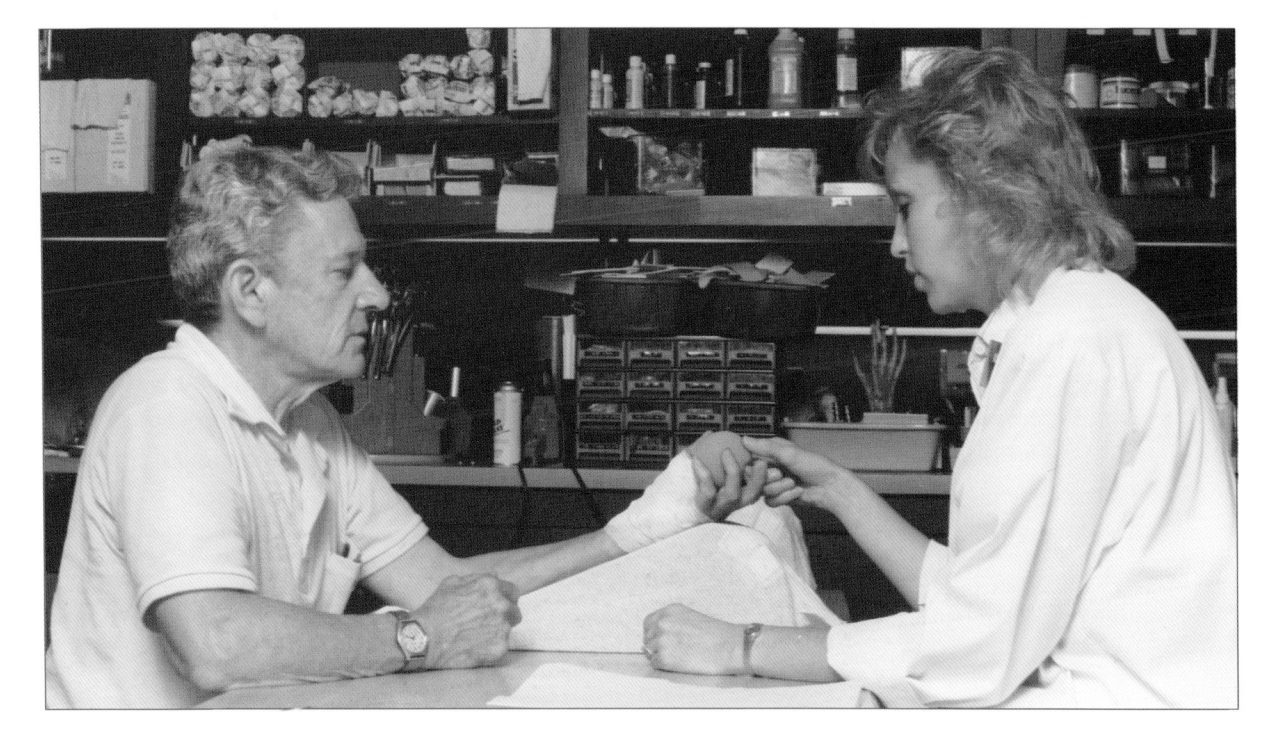

Along with Dr. David Larson, department chair, this group of plastic and reconstructive surgeons also introduced free flap surgery within the state. With this procedure, doctors remove a section of skin, underlying tissue, and small stubs of a vein, artery, and nerve from one area of the body, such as the back of the upper arm. They then reattach this free flap to the existing arteries, veins, and nerves of the injured area in another section of the body. A similar procedure is utilized in breast reconstruction following mastectomies. Dr. Larson was one of the first in the state's medical history to perform this tran-abdominal procedure.

Other new technologies in Froedtert's early years included new diagnostic procedures with nuclear magnetic resonance that were especially valuable for spinal cord and neurological disorders.

In 1982, the General Clinical Research Center moved into Froedtert Hospital. It was the only research center affiliated with a medical school in Wisconsin and one of only seventy-five in the country. It helped to attract trained physicians with outstanding academic credentials. This, in turn, helped strengthen the quality of clinical teaching and increase the body of knowledge for a variety of disorders.

Gastroenterology physicians and hospital technicians invented several instruments crucial to diagnosing esophageal and gastric problems. No fewer than five of these inventions are now used by gastroenterologists worldwide. Gastroenterologists and otolaryngologists combined their clinical research efforts to develop diagnostic procedures and therapies for patients with swallowing disorders. This multi-specialty effort led to the founding of the Dysphagia Institute. The Institute has become a major resource for physicians throughout the world in caring for patients with swallowing disorders.

Otolaryngologists pioneered laser surgery for ear, nose, and throat problems. Surgeons used lasers to evaporate tumors in the larynx and taught other surgeons from around the country the procedure. The state's first cochlear implant surgery to restore sound to the hearing impaired was performed at Froedtert.

Medical College urologists and the hospital's biomedical engineering staff developed the country's first computerized urodynamic instrumentation to measure urinary flow. When the hospital was designated as one of only three prostate centers in the country, Froedtert purchased equipment that utilized laser surgery as a less invasive procedure to reduce enlarged prostate glands. Microscopic equipment in surgery enabled hospital staff to develop a number of extraordinary procedures in neurosurgery and in plastic and reconstructive surgery that were previously unavailable in this area of the state.

Dr. Mark Adams, director of Transplant Surgery, performed the state's first liver transplant in early September of

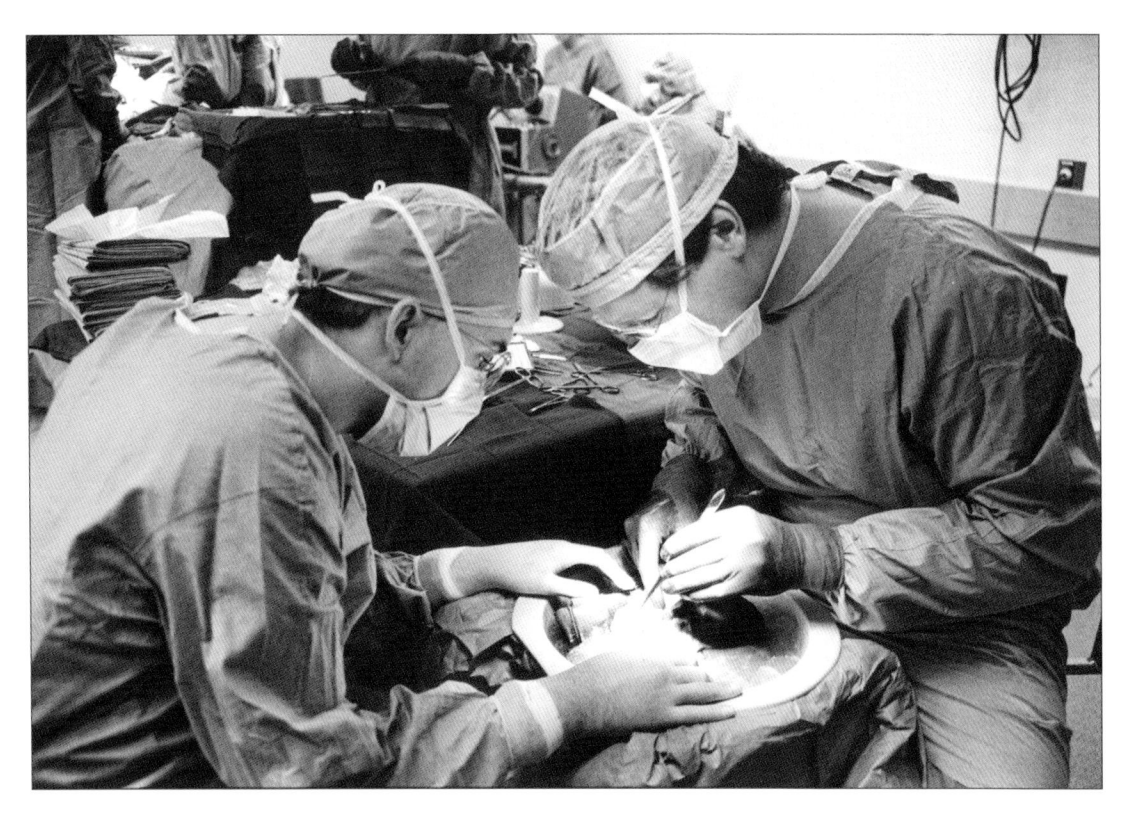

Doctors performing a pancreas transplant in 1992

1983—a year that could be classified as the beginning of a turnaround for Froedtert hospital. By 1985, the hospital was performing scores of kidney transplants and multiple liver transplants annually. In 2006, 247 heart, lung, kidney, liver, pancreas, blood, and bone and marrow transplants were performed.

In partnership with the Zablocki Veteran's Hospital, Froedtert became the first hospital in the state to utilize shock wave therapy as a noninvasive method to crush painful kidney stones. This unique partnership between a private and federal hospital to provide a consolidated service was questioned by local health planners, but Froedtert and the VA prevailed and the service began operations in 1983. A unique clinical teaching program in shock wave therapy was initiated by Froedtert's urologists. Private practice physicians admitted their patients to Froedtert and then learned the techniques by participating in the procedure with Froedtert urologists. In time, when shock wave therapy instrumentation was made available in their respective communities, they had the knowledge and skill to provide the service. ■

Chapter 30

Changing the Face of Healthcare

As Froedtert and the Medical College's reputation grew, so did the financial woes of the venerable Milwaukee County Medical Complex. Milwaukee County was well aware of the difficulty of maintaining effective hospital operations under the burden of the cumbersome multi-committee approval processes of the County Board. The structure had threatened the creation of the Milwaukee Regional Medical Center itself in the 1960s and 1970s, and it continued to create the same havoc in the 1980s and 1990s for Milwaukee County Hospital, by then known as the Milwaukee County Medical Complex.

A series of studies on the governance structure for the County Medical Complex began as early as 1977. Conducted at different times and under different circumstances, each of the eleven studies differed in some details but in each instance recommended significant changes be made with regard to the governance and administration of the hospital. Consistent in those recommendations was the need to place broad administrative responsibilities in the hands of professional administrators while limiting the role of County government to final approval of general policy and budgets. For the most part, those studies languished in the mire of County bureaucracy and went nowhere.

In 1985, Froedtert Hospital and the Milwaukee County Medical Complex jointly commissioned a study by Robert Douglass Associates to identify an organizational structure that would allow them to compete more effectively in the healthcare marketplace while maintaining their missions of quality patient care, teaching, research, and community service. The Douglass Report, issued in July of that year, recommended the establishment of a non-profit corporation that would independently contract with Milwaukee County Hospital and Froedtert Memorial Lutheran Hospital to jointly manage and operate the programs, services, and workforces of both organizations.

A joint management resolution setting forth the principal findings of the Douglass Report went to the County Board and was recommended for inclusion in the

1986 Milwaukee County Executive Budget. The resolution was submitted with endorsements from the boards of Froedtert Hospital, the Medical College of Wisconsin, Curative Rehabilitation Center, the Blood Center of Wisconsin, Children's Hospital, and the Milwaukee Regional Medical Center. The resolution, passed by the County Board, called for the formation of a Joint Management Committee to oversee a task force. It was charged with establishing the framework for a joint management corporation. However, in order to proceed, Milwaukee County needed a change in state legislation to contract with a non-profit corporation rather than operate the hospital itself as required by existing statutes.

In the meantime, the Medical Complex continued to struggle, unable to respond effectively to the competitive marketplace of the 1980s. A flawed patient accounts system added to the problems, and by 1989 the Milwaukee County Medical Complex was in crisis, projecting a $12 to $18 million deficit and carrying over $57 million in accounts receivable. Once the Complex's deficit became public, Howard Fuller, then director of the County's Health and Human Services Programs, fired County Hospital Administrator William I. Jenkins. In November 1989, Mary Julia (Julie) Hanser, former president and CEO of St. Mary's Hospital in Milwaukee, was named to replace Jenkins.

This growing fiscal crisis for Milwaukee County Hospital did not bode well for Froedtert. Given the interdependency of the two hospitals, the financial volatility of County Hospital had the potential to threaten the financial stability of Froedtert and the Medical College as well. And the Douglass Report seemed to have gone the way of other studies before it. No definitive answer to respond to the crisis was on the table.

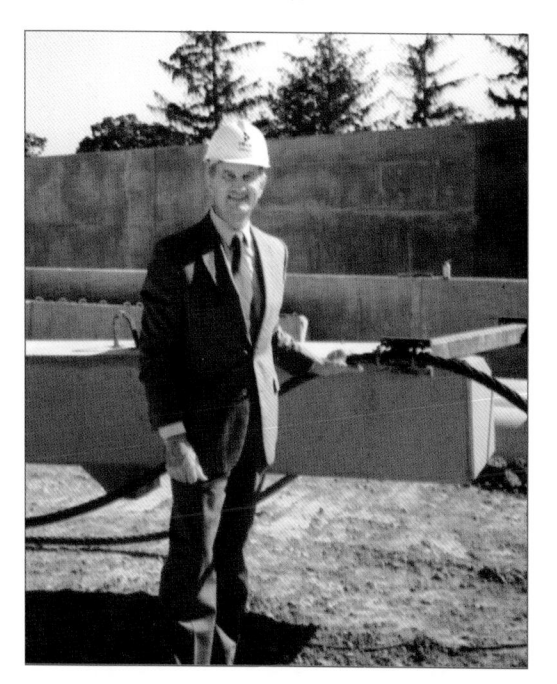

While the Milwaukee County Medical Complex was experiencing problems, Froedtert continued to expand. Wearing a hard hat, Froedtert President and CEO Dean Roe inspects the West Clinics construction site.

To get the ball rolling, County Supervisor Susan Baldwin called for yet another study. Released in April 1990, it essentially supported an earlier September 1988 County Board staff study by recommending that the Medical Complex become an independent department of County government, run by a board of directors.

According to Supervisor Baldwin, the bottom-line goal was to reduce the hospital's dependence on the County's tax levy. The report was endorsed by the *Business Journal*, the *Milwaukee Journal*, and the *Milwaukee Sentinel* as it made its way through the Health and Finance Committees and to the County Board.

While the creation of County Hospital as an independent department appeared to have support from most Milwaukee County officials, the idea of a separate board overseeing the operations and finances faced strong opposition on many fronts. Supervisors Terrance Pitts and Elizabeth Coggs-Jones, with support from the Black Health Coalition, argued that a separate board would reduce its accountability to County officials and its dedication to caring for the poor. Pitts, as chair of the Health Committee, was reluctant to give up jurisdiction until these concerns were resolved. Former County Executive John Doyne, County Board Chairman F. Thomas Ament, and County Supervisor Robert Jackson feared that a separate board only added to the bureaucracy.

In the end, a compromise resolution was approved by the County Board. It recommended that the hospital be established as a separate County agency with a study panel to work out the details of running it. Like the studies and recommendations before it, this "Blue Ribbon Committee" resolution seemed to fade from the radar screen after passage. Interestingly, however, it was in the Blue Ribbon debate that the seeds of dramatic change were first planted by Supervisor Robert Jackson when he publicly suggested it might be in the County's best interest to get out of the hospital business.

In February 1991, the Greater Milwaukee Committee entered the picture and moved the discussion back into focus by announcing that it would conduct its own study on the future of the Milwaukee County Medical Complex. Its report, released in July of that year, went a little farther than the Blue Ribbon study. It called for a public-private partnership with an independent board of directors that would contract with Milwaukee County to govern the Medical Complex with the management control to separately operate the hospital. The hospital would continue to own the assets, but it would be managed by the independent board.

While the GMC study was going on, Supervisor Daniel Casey fueled Bob Jackson's position by proposing to privatize the Medical Complex and write off its operating debt of $60 million to Milwaukee County by January 1992. His proposal called for a transition team to negotiate a transfer of the Medical Complex's operations to either Froedtert Hospital, a consortium of Milwaukee Regional Medical Center members, or a private non-profit entity. The Casey resolution stalled in the Health Committee. ■

Chapter 31

Gale-Force Winds of Change Begin a New Era

That was the landscape when Froedtert President Dean Roe announced his retirement in 1992. Roe had presided over the creation of Froedtert, a tumultuous process that took over thirty years to its opening in September 1980. He was leaving a hospital that under his leadership had already achieved significant recognition as an academic hospital offering innovative treatments and programs.

About the same time, Julie Hanser, who had managed to stabilize the Medical Complex and see it through the opening of its Ambulatory Care Center and name change to John L. Doyne Hospital, announced her resignation to take a position as president and CEO of Mercy Health Partners of Southwest Ohio.

With leadership changing at both of its major teaching hospitals and frustrated by the lack of action on the governance of County Hospital, now John L. Doyne Hospital, the Medical College of Wisconsin Board approved a resolution calling for the creation of a single adult hospital on the grounds of the Milwaukee Regional Medical Center. That was January 1993.

One month later, Roe's successor, William Petasnick, arrived on campus and the winds of change began to blow hard and steady. Petasnick was a Wisconsin native, born and raised in Sheboygan, and his career had begun in Wisconsin. In a twist of fate, in 1976, while he was a member of senior management at the University of Wisconsin Hospital and Clinics, he was asked to do a review of the Froedtert Hospital application by the Wisconsin Division of Health Policy and Planning.

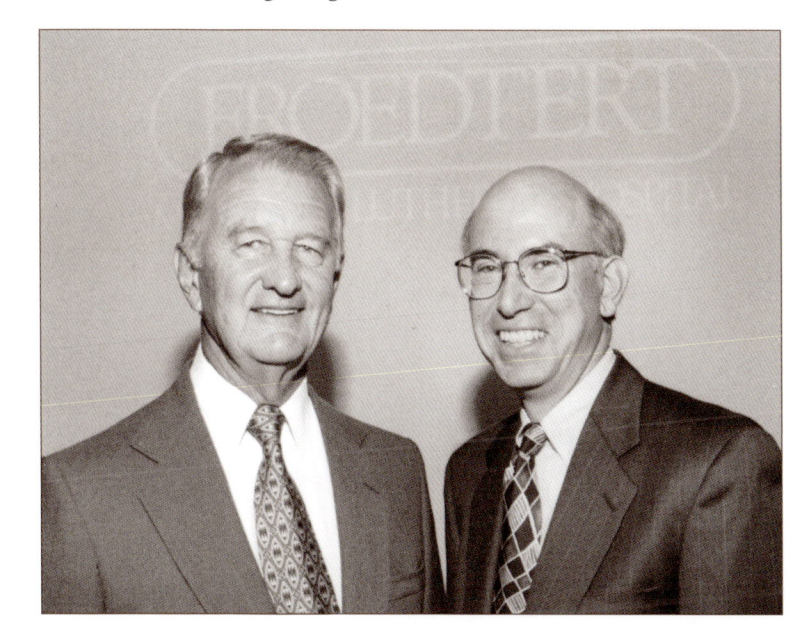

Dean Roe (left) was Froedtert Hospital's first president. William Petasnick took over the helm in February 1993 and continues to serve today.

125

William D. Petasnick, Froedtert's President and CEO

William D. Petasnick assumed the role of President and CEO of Froedtert Hospital in 1993, only the second president and CEO in the hospital's history. When he arrived, Froedtert had already achieved recognition as a strong teaching hospital under his predecessor, Dean Roe.

It was up to Petasnick to ensure that Froedtert Hospital became a true academic medical center. And he did so with blinding speed. By the end of 1995, Froedtert Hospital swelled from 241 to 473 staffed beds, increased staff from 1,325 to 2,100, and more than doubled annual operating revenue when County General Hospital closed and Froedtert assumed all of its programs and services. Petasnick provided the skilled leadership that allowed this monumental event to happen without a blip in the continuum of care for patients. In less than two years, he had taken Froedtert Hospital from a strong teaching hospital to Southeastern Wisconsin's only adult academic medical center. And that was just the beginning.

By 2006, the American Hospital Association named William D. Petasnick its chairman-elect. He had emerged as a national leader from the strength and character of his leadership at Froedtert. In less than twelve years, Froedtert had achieved state and national recognition on a variety of fronts. The CEO shepherded the partnership that in 2001 created Froedtert & Community Health System, an integrated health system between Froedtert Hospital and Community Memorial Hospital. He became known statewide for his collaborative approach with other providers. His focus was on ensuring that patients received the right care, at the right time, and in the right facility. He forged partnerships that strengthened services in local communities while improving access to Froedtert's tertiary care programs. Those partnerships include United Hospital System in Kenosha, ThedaCare and Agnesian Health in the Fox Valley, and Bellin Health in Green Bay.

Under his leadership, Froedtert received national recognition for excellence in healthcare services. He focused on improving healthcare quality while holding the line on costs, moving Froedtert from a position of average charge per case that was 31 percent above the market in 1996, to 12 percent below the market average by the end of 2006. His drive for quality led Froedtert to become one of the first hospitals in the nation to apply Six Sigma methodology to reduce medical errors. The hospital was also a founding member of the Wisconsin Collaborative for Healthcare Quality.

Prior to being named president of Froedtert Hospital, Petasnick served as the administrator and chief operating officer of the University of Iowa Hospital and Clinics. He also held senior management positions at the University of North Carolina Hospital at Chapel Hill and the University of Wisconsin Hospital and Clinics.

Petasnick has been involved in numerous national, statewide, and regional committees, including a three-year term on the Board of Trustees of the American Hospital Association, Chair of the Council of Teaching Hospitals and Health Systems for the Association of American Medical Colleges, and a member of the Board of Directors of the University HealthSystem Consortium. He is a past chairman of the Wisconsin Hospital Association. He is also a member of the Greater Milwaukee Committee and serves on the board of the BloodCenter of Wisconsin. He is a member of the Downtown Rotary Club and several other civic organizations. Petasnick also serves on the Board of Directors of the Metropolitan Milwaukee Association of Commerce.

Petasnick received a bachelor's degree from the University of Wisconsin and a master's degree in hospital and healthcare administration from the University of Minnesota. In 2007, Petasnick was awarded an honorary doctorate degree from the University of Wisconsin-Milwaukee.

He recalled leaving the state to become the chief operating officer at the University of North Carolina Hospital at Chapel Hill, not knowing if Froedtert Hospital was ever built. He was coming to Milwaukee from his position as administrator and chief operating officer of the University of Iowa Hospital and Clinics, a well-established academic medical center. To Petasnick, the dysfunction between Froedtert and Doyne was a challenge. As he explained, "I saw the opportunity to create something unique and an unfulfilled vision that needed to be achieved." He knew the history, and it was clear upon his arrival that the two organizations needed to quickly find solutions together or neither was going to survive.

He arrived just before Hanser's departure, so they were unable to move an agenda forward together. She was only able to bring Petasnick up to date on governance discussions and share copies of the many studies that had been completed since 1977. And then she was gone.

As luck would have it, just as Petasnick was wading through the many studies, John R. Petersen, MD, former medical director at Doyne Hospital, was named interim administrator until a replacement for Hanser could be found. Petersen knew every study intimately, having been a part of it all in his role as medical director at the hospital. He was well known and well respected throughout Milwaukee County and was in a unique position to bring influence and credibility to any discussions about joint solutions.

By March 1993, Petersen and Petasnick had begun informal discussions about ways to create a unified approach to patient care that would work in the marketplace and be in the best interest of the patients and community. It was that theme of "in the best interest of the patients and community" that linked these two from their first meeting. Petasnick remembered that meeting as one in which "I could tell that John's heart and soul were at County Hospital, but even more strongly that they were tied to the community and serving the patient, especially the uninsured. We were on same field, ready to play the same game. We both knew we had to get beyond the politics and find what would be best for the community."

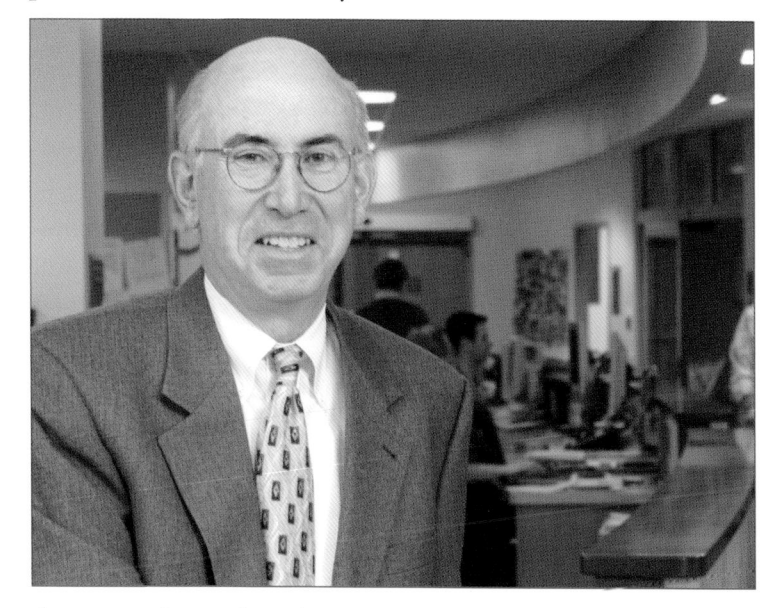

Bill Petasnick, Froedtert's President and CEO since 1993

They committed themselves to detailed discussions about how they could redefine the partnership between the two hospitals. They brought in consultants to help assess the situation in light of the new competitive environment sweeping the country. By September, they had gathered enough information. They assembled briefing books that clearly and concisely articulated the challenges facing the two hospitals, their poor position in the marketplace in terms of costs and revenues, and the potential benefits from the perspective of patients that could be derived from the creation of a single hospital. They cited cost savings and revenue enhancements that could be generated through a model similar to the joint venture recommended in the Douglass study of 1985. Together they began to quietly meet with county and community leaders, sharing their briefing books and engaging in meaningful dialogue about what it would take to best serve the community.

One of those first meetings was a briefing for T. Michael Bolger, president of the Medical College of Wisconsin; James Keyes, chair of the Medical College Board; and County Executive F. Thomas Ament. Keyes and Bolger were already on record regarding a single adult hospital, but the hope was to engage Ament. In the course of that meeting, Ament indicated his support of a "singular" hospital concept, but cautioned that it would take incremental steps.

By October, Ament, Petasnick, and Petersen had reached agreement to form a hospital consolidation working group that would include themselves as well as Bolger; Thomas Smallwood, the chair of the Froedtert Board; a County Board supervisor; and Keyes, representing the Greater Milwaukee Committee. Robert Jackson, County Board chair, was targeted for the supervisor slot. Jackson was briefed and, while supportive, raised his concern once again that maybe it was time for the County to get out of the hospital business.

In late November, the entire group, including Jackson, met and finalized the details of a process and work group charged to identify and analyze organizational options for creating a single hospital. Recommendations on a preferred option were to be ready for presentation by March 31, 1994. Immediately the behind-the-scenes work intensified.

At the same time, efforts to recruit a new Doyne Hospital administrator continued. In a somewhat controversial move, County Executive Ament nominated Terrence M. Hansen, former head of Cook County Hospital in Chicago. This was over the objections of the Selection Committee and some County Board supervisors, who questioned Hansen's qualifications. Charges flew that Hansen was more of a politician than a hospital manager and that controlling the finances of Doyne required tight management. Creating more anxiety in the midst of the Hansen controversy was another call by Bob Jackson to get the County out of the hospital business. In the end, Hansen's appointment was approved by the County Board.

March 1994 saw an emergence of a number of events that set the stage for formalizing the Doyne-Froedtert discussions. To begin with, John L. Doyne Hospital was back in the red and back in the news, reporting deficits nearing $5 million. Then, a state statute change, sparked by the 1985 Douglass study, was finally signed by the governor. The change gave Milwaukee County the authority to contract with a non-profit board to manage its hospital. Next, Terrence Hansen went public saying Doyne was discussing an alliance with Froedtert and considering joining Horizon Healthcare, Inc., a collaborative hospital system that included Froedtert, Columbia, Community Memorial of Menomonee Falls, St. Mary's, St. Mary's-Ozaukee, and St. Mary's Hill hospitals, and Seton Health Corporation of Wisconsin. While out of step with the behind-the-scenes discussions, Hansen's public statements did reflect some elements of the options emerging from the work group for a new combined structure for Froedtert and Doyne. Finally, Supervisor Lee Holloway, chair of the County Board's Health Committee, was brought into the briefing circle, and he and Jackson became key to formalizing the process.

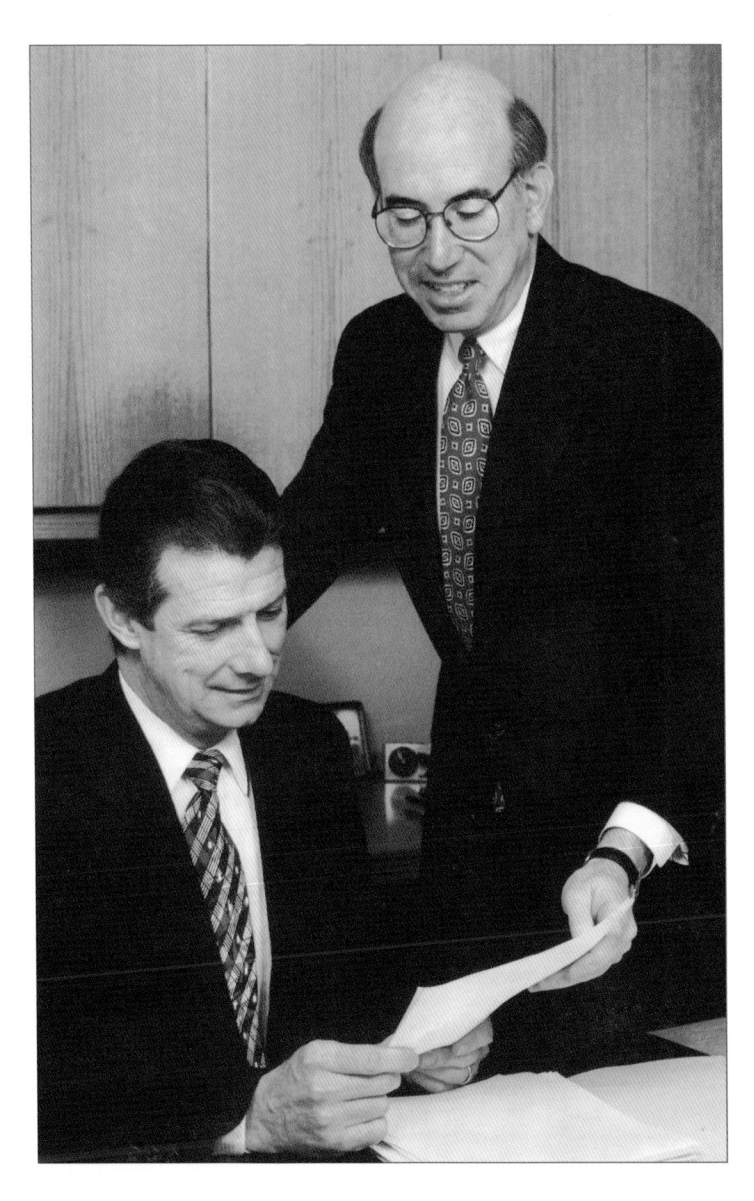

By mid-April, Milwaukee County and Froedtert Hospital had executed a Memorandum of Understanding to achieve a definitive agreement for implementing a new joint operating structure for Froedtert and Doyne. A key element was "a structure that would operate as a *non-governmental*

Thomas Smallwood (left), Froedtert Board Chairman from 1985 until 2001, and Froedtert President and CEO Bill Petasnick

organization." The memorandum called for a series of steps leading to a new corporate entity and joint operations beginning by January 1, 1995. Those timelines turned out to be off by almost exactly one year.

A working committee led by Petasnick, Hansen, and Petersen began meeting immediately, but discussions seemed to flounder due to external pressures on Hansen. In July, the group was forced to ask for an extension of the timeline. It took until early September for its preliminary report to be ready; the report recommended that a new non-governmental parent corporation be formed to manage and control the assets of both Froedtert and Doyne hospitals. At that point, and with the viability of Doyne Hospital seeming even more fragile, two more key County Supervisors, Karen Ordinans and Lynne DeBruin, were briefed on the issues and status of the discussions. They quickly immersed themselves in the process and joined Jackson and Holloway in driving decisions that would be in the best interest of the community.

Turmoil continued at John L. Doyne Hospital. By late September, Ament bowed to pressure and Terrence Hansen was replaced by Interim Administrator Thomas Brophy, who was tapped from his job as director of Human Services for Milwaukee County.

Within days of arriving at Doyne Hospital, Brophy was at Petasnick's door, shaking his head and wondering how Doyne was going to survive based on his initial appraisal of the situation. Petasnick had a briefing book ready and quickly brought Brophy up to speed on the work group recommendations. Brophy left that day determined to see things move quickly. Ordinans, Jackson, DeBruin, and Holloway then took the lead in moving forward a key resolution that passed the County Board in October. That resolution called for establishing a work group to develop a definitive agreement with Froedtert to create a single non-governmental, adult, acute care hospital.

In December 1994, the County Board of Supervisors approved a definitive agreement with Froedtert Hospital to enter into negotiations for the development of a detailed implementation plan for one adult, acute care hospital to be achieved through either the "creation of a new, non-governmental entity to manage and control the combined assets and programs of Doyne and Froedtert" or "consideration of alternative plans for the transfer of Doyne assets including a direct sale or long-term lease." That second clause was pivotal as negotiations moved forward.

The negotiating team included the original work group along with attorneys for Froedtert and Corporation Counsel for Milwaukee County; William Drew, director of Administration for the County and a close ally of Tom Ament; and Blaine O'Connell, Froedtert's Chief Financial Officer. The negotiating team initiated a joint Doyne and Froedtert financial feasibility study conducted by outside consultants, a study that encompassed financial projections of the options under consideration, as well as the status quo. This proved to be an extremely critical piece in the process and led to an outcome that no one would have predicted when all this began in 1993. The results showed that Milwaukee County could anticipate ongoing operating deficits and negative cash balances that would translate into overall County support for Doyne Hospital reaching $51.9 million by the year 2000. It became abundantly clear to the negotiating team that Milwaukee County needed to get out of the hospital business if it wished to avoid financial disaster.

But as strong as the financial arguments might be, the negotiating team recognized that there was equally strong emotional attachment to the hospital on many fronts, emotions that could easily cloud the reality of the numbers. So in March, before any recommendations were formally presented to the County Board, Ament, Jackson, and Holloway invited all the County supervisors to attend a half-day session on national health trends. They stressed the importance of attendance "given the magnitude of the policy issues facing Milwaukee County government as we consider the future of Doyne Hospital." All twenty-five supervisors, along with staff from the County Board and County Executive's office and the negotiating team,

attended the presentation. Robert J. Baker, president of the national University Hospital Consortium, was the keynote speaker. He presented information about the challenges and market forces facing healthcare providers across the country, particularly those affiliated with academic medical centers. His presentation made it clear that public hospitals across the country were under extreme stress and many were being forced to close, sometimes without good contingency plans in place for a continuum of care for patients.

Then Brophy and Petasnick outlined the findings of the feasibility study and an extensive market analysis that clearly showed the precarious position of both hospitals. They then reported some of the conclusions being reached by the negotiating team. Their report was sobering and at the same time enlightening, and it seemed to move even the strongest supporters of the hospital to acknowledge that alternatives needed to be considered.

That paved the way for the County Board's Health and Finance Committees to accept the recommendations presented by the negotiating team. The two primary recommendations were: (1) Two adult hospitals were not financially feasible, and (2) Milwaukee County needed to discontinue its role as a direct provider and assume a new role as a purchaser of services.

On April 13, 1995, the County Board of Supervisors, in a landmark vote, approved discontinuing the County's role as a direct provider of medical services and terminating operation of Doyne Hospital, effective no later than December 31, 1995. Simultaneously the County Board called for negotiations with Froedtert Hospital for the purchase or long-term lease of Doyne Hospital's assets.

By September 7, 1995, Milwaukee County approved the terms and conditions of a binding agreement between Milwaukee County and Froedtert Hospital. Key provisions of the agreement included:

- Milwaukee County would discontinue its role as a direct provider of medical services and terminate its operation of Doyne Hospital by December 31, 1995,
- Milwaukee County would contract with Froedtert to provide services through an interim services agreement until the closure of Doyne Hospital,
- Froedtert Hospital would purchase Doyne Hospital assets from Milwaukee County,
- Milwaukee County would amend Froedtert's existing land lease to include the Doyne Hospital land,
- Froedtert would remain a preferred provider to the General Assistance–Medical Program (GA-MP) for two years, and
- Froedtert would maintain an Emergency Department and Level 1 Trauma Center for two years.

Now the negotiating team was faced with hammering out all the details to bring those provisions to reality. It was a daunting challenge that needed to be accomplished in about three months. On December 20, 1995, one day before the planned closing of Doyne Hospital, the final documents were signed by Froedtert and Milwaukee County. It took five three-inch binders to hold the legal documents that defined every aspect of this very complicated deal that had taken two years to achieve.

The make-or-break aspects of the deal centered around three key issues: the sale or lease price, transitional funding for indigent care, and the environmental risks associated with the Doyne Hospital buildings.

Initially the two parties were miles apart on price. Froedtert determined the value of the Doyne Hospital physical plant based on the revenue to be generated from business that could be located in those buildings; in contrast, Milwaukee County looked at the current debt obligations associated with the facility and at what it perceived to be its fair market value. In the end, the two parties reached a creative off-balance-sheet solution that included a relatively modest up-front payment of $4.1 million for the Doyne assets and a lease of the associated land based on a percentage of positive operating cash flow for twenty-five years. It was a win-win solution. Froedtert's debt levels would not be impacted, and Milwaukee County had the potential to receive significant revenue dependent upon Froedtert's success.

Transitional funding for indigent care was the simplest of the key issues to resolve, since GA-MP dollars were an existing part of the County's budget, put in place years earlier as a way to track monies spent to care for the uninsured in Milwaukee County separate from the cost of operating the hospital. Along with the funding and Froedtert's commitment to serve as the preferred provider for GA-MP for two years, Froedtert also agreed to assume a leadership role in developing a community-based primary care network for underserved residents eligible for GA-MP.

The numerous environmental problems in the older portions of Doyne Hospital, ranging from asbestos in the walls and ceilings to mercury in the piping system, created the most complex aspect of the negotiations. In the end, Milwaukee County accepted liability associated with those factors, including assuming responsibility for all environmental costs involved in any future demolition of the buildings. In addition, while Froedtert bought the buildings, the effluent water and sewer systems remained the property of Milwaukee County. As a final precaution, Froedtert

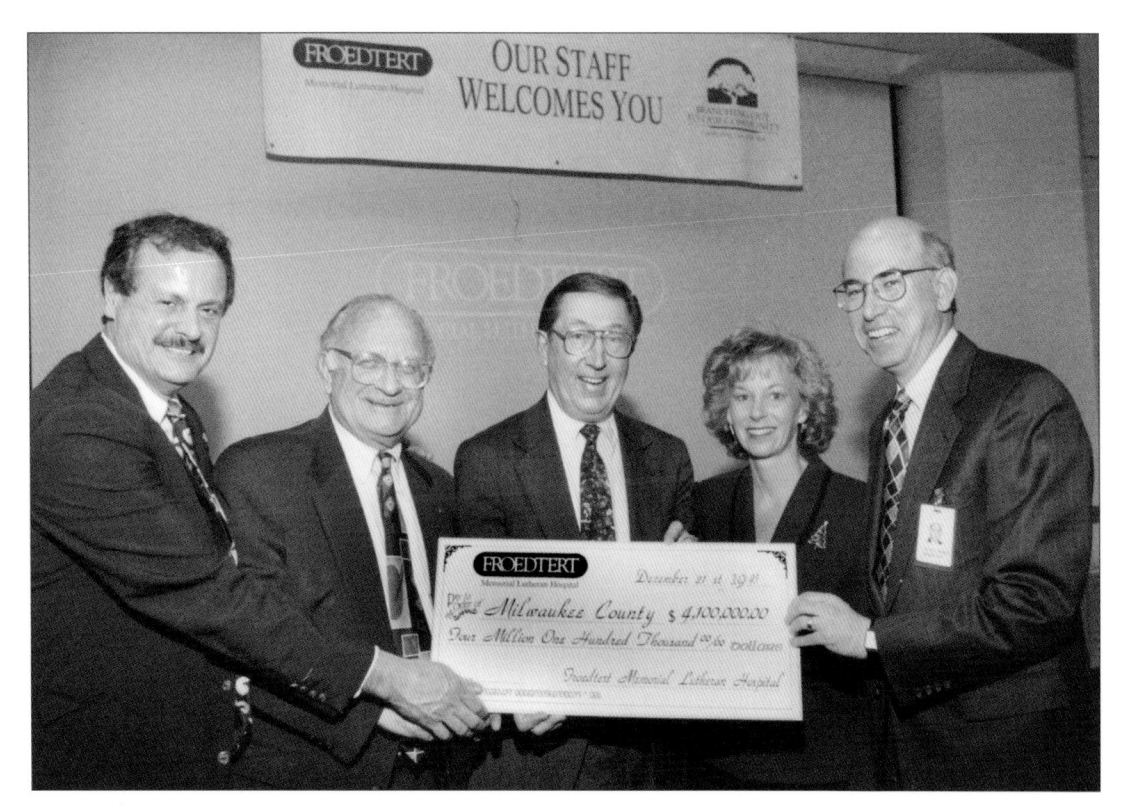

Froedtert President and CEO Bill Petasnick (far right) presents a check for $4.1 million to Milwaukee County officials for the purchase of Doyne Hospital.

also obtained waivers from appropriate governmental entities insulating it from any future claims.

Brophy described it all as "... a long and difficult process, that led to what I believe was a monumental policy decision made in the best interest of patients and taxpayers in the community." He credited the success of the efforts to "negotiating teams made up of top-notch, quality people

The Medical College of Wisconsin

The Medical College of Wisconsin traces its history back to 1893 with the founding of both the Wisconsin College of Physicians and Surgeons and the Milwaukee Medical College. The Milwaukee Medical College was absorbed by Marquette University in 1907, becoming a department within the university. It wasn't until the Wisconsin College of Physicians and Surgeons merged with the Milwaukee Medical College on January 14, 1913, that Marquette established a School of Medicine, the Marquette University School of Medicine.

After World War II, Marquette University School of Medicine, like its counterparts nationally, was asked to affiliate with Milwaukee's Veterans Administration Medical Center. This was being done nationwide to upgrade the quality of medicine provided to returning war veterans. Nothing came of that request.

During the 1950s and 1960s, the school was plagued by financial difficulties, a source of great concern to Marquette University. On September 30, 1967, Marquette University terminated its sponsorship of the medical school. A private, freestanding institution under the name Marquette School of Medicine was established. The medical school's board of directors determined that the medical school provided statewide services and should be named to reflect its ties to all residents of Wisconsin. On October 14, 1970, the medical school was renamed the Medical College of Wisconsin.

The Medical College of Wisconsin began a period of extraordinary growth in 1978 when it moved to its new facilities on the campus of the Milwaukee Regional Medical Center. After establishing itself as a major referral center for tertiary care, the Medical College introduced new initiatives, including an emphasis on primary care and outpatient services, programs in inner city and rural areas, establishment of Centers of Excellence, and growth of the Graduate School of Biomedical Sciences. The Medical College, to date, has established more than thirty urban initiatives focused on a wide range of public health issues.

Between 1986 and 2007, on-campus construction was seemingly nonstop. The Medical College added the MACC Fund Research Center; the Medical College Clinics at Froedtert; a fourth-floor addition to the Medical Education Building; and, in the fall of 1998, the Health Research Center, the new "front door" to the College. The $36 million Health Research Center focuses in large part on medical informatics and genetic research. In January 2007, the Medical College and Children's Hospital Health System opened the new $117 million Translational and Biomedical Research Center/Children's Research Institute.

In 2006, the college reported an enrollment of 1,359 students, including 805 medical students and 554 graduate students as well as physicians in the Master of Public Health Degree program. More than 1,100 faculty physicians provide adult and pediatric care to more than 260,000 patients, representing more than one million patient visits annually.

A major national research center, the Medical College of Wisconsin and its faculty received $123 million in external support for research and training. In 2004, it was ranked forty-second among the nation's top medical schools for National Institutes of Health research funding, placing the college in the top one-third of the nation's 125 medical schools. The faculty conducts more than 1,500 research studies annually in all areas of medicine.

who trusted each other, didn't play games, put things on the table straight forward, and put aside controversial issues until creative approaches could be found." Equally important, according to Brophy, was the ability to have good people to continue to run Doyne Hospital while the closure negotiations were ongoing. He credited Paula Lucey, who was serving as associate administrator for Patient Care Services, and Charlie Runge, an assistant administrator, for keeping those day-to-day operations moving smoothly and maintaining high quality of care. Both Lucey and Runge emerged as continuing leaders after the transition. Lucey went on to work for Milwaukee County to lead the redesign and implementation of the community-based GA-MP program. Runge became a vice president at Froedtert, leading the evolution and growth of the clinical services in cooperation with the Medical College.

At midnight on December 21, 1995, a metamorphosis of sorts took place. Milwaukee County ended 135 years of directly providing medical services to its citizens and became a purchaser of services. Simultaneously Froedtert Hospital expanded its program and services. It was a monumental moment that came and went very quietly and without a blip in the continuum of care for patients. Overnight Froedtert swelled from 241 to 473 staffed beds; hospital staff increased from 1,325 to 2,100; and annual operating revenue more than doubled, from $159 million to $325 million.

Now all medical services were together as Cardiovascular, Cancer, Musculoskeletal, Emergency & Trauma, and Women's Health Center services moved to Froedtert Hospital. After thirty years of twists and turns, study after study, controversy, politics, and compromise, Froedtert Hospital emerged as Southeastern Wisconsin's only adult academic medical center.

The 135-year-old roots of Milwaukee County's hospital, Froedtert's youthful energy, and the medical expertise of the Medical College of Wisconsin physicians combined to create a new leader poised for greatness. Indeed, it was just the beginning of a story of medical breakthroughs, nationally recognized services, and multiple successes and achievements for Froedtert Hospital, an academic medical center grounded and formed "in the best interest of the patient." ∎

Epilogue

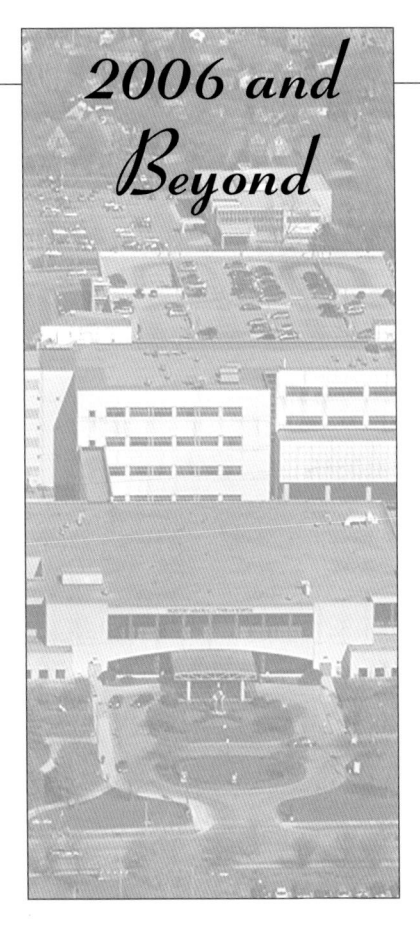

2006 and Beyond

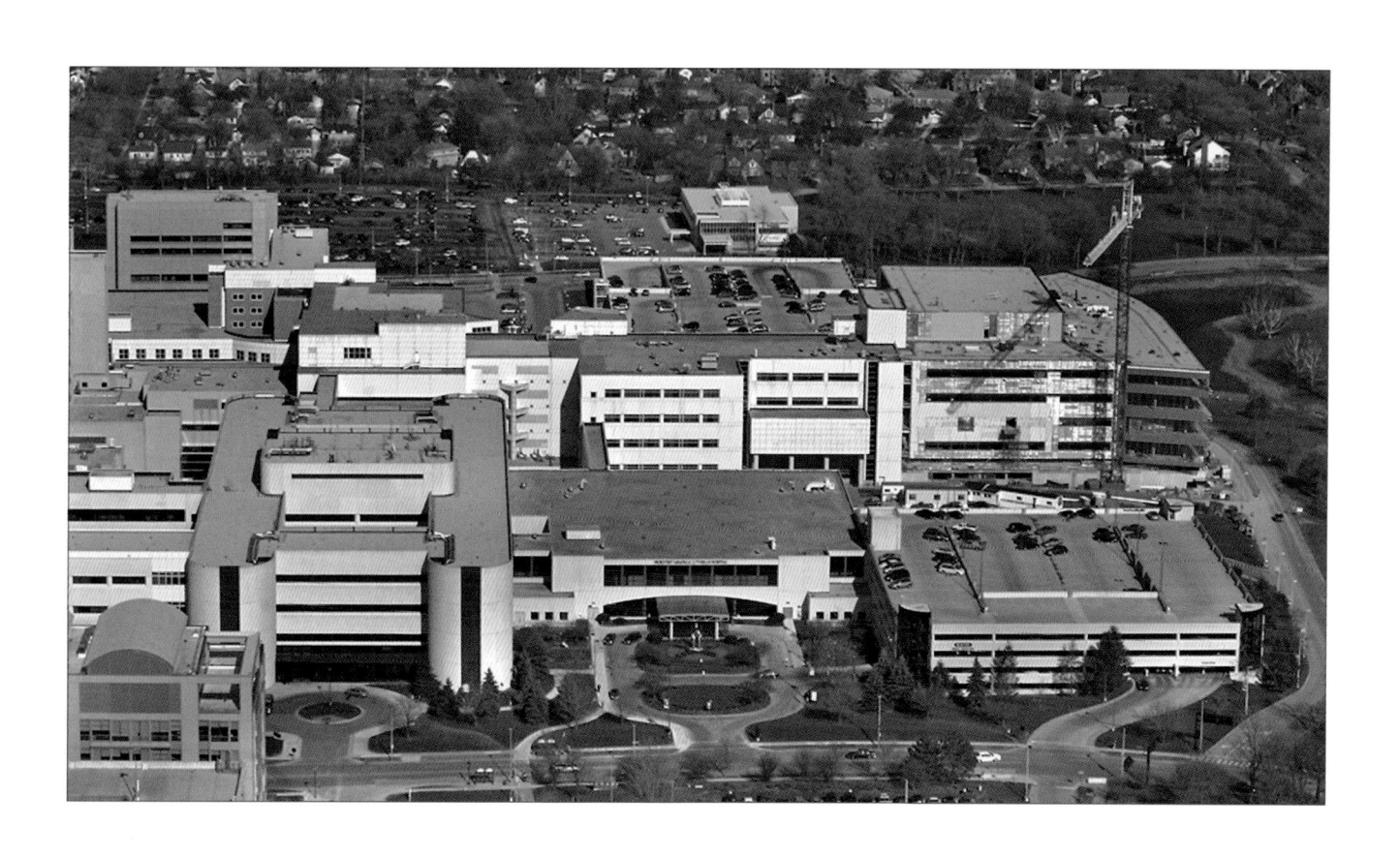

And the Whirlwind Continues

In November 1996, a feature article about Bill Petasnick guiding Froedtert Hospital past the closure of Doyne appeared in the *Business Journal Serving Greater Milwaukee*. The headline read, "Change, Change, Change," a clear indication of the whirlwind that would be created by this emerging academic medical center. By the time it reached its twenty-fifth birthday in September 2005, Froedtert Hospital had achieved remarkable growth and success. That year, 23,617 patients were admitted to Froedtert, and the hospital tallied 454,780 outpatient visits. Petasnick and his team had taken Froedtert on a rapid ride of medical advances and business achievements. These achievements encompassed a wide range of areas.

In 1993, Froedtert, along with the Medical College of Wisconsin, was named one of two world sites for the clinical evaluation of advanced radiology and imaging systems.

The Neurosurgical and Radiology staff, working with GE Medical Systems, pioneered new computer graphics techniques converting two-dimensional CT images into three-dimensional pictures. Using this new technology, neurosurgeons could view three-dimensional interior and exterior images of, for example, the skull for preoperative planning. This technology was a major benefit to the neurosurgeons as well as the patient undergoing cranial and other neurosurgical procedures.

In 1996, Froedtert Hospital became a comprehensive center for all types of transplantation services as bone marrow and heart and lung transplantation programs were added to existing kidney, liver, and pancreas programs. By 1997, more than two thousand kidney transplants had been performed at the hospital. The program was declared one of the nation's twenty largest centers for kidney transplantation. That year, the state's first bone marrow transplant for severe progressive multiple sclerosis was performed at Froedtert—it was the second such surgery in the nation. A rare double-lung transplant on a cystic fibrosis patient was also done in 1997. In 2002, an uncommon piggyback liver transplant was performed by attaching a donor liver to the patient's own liver. By 2003, Froedtert was the seventeenth most active kidney transplant program in the country,

(opposite page) Froedtert Hospital, 2007

with more than three thousand performed since the program began in 1967.

The 2006 Froedtert Annual Report revealed that the organ transplantation program was still incredibly active with 124 kidney, 30 liver, 8 pancreas, 4 lung, and 2 heart transplants done that year. Additionally, 79 blood and marrow transplants were performed in 2006.

In addition to establishing a national reputation for transplantation, Froedtert has continued to build its reputation in leading-edge cancer care.

Froedtert & the Medical College of Wisconsin Cancer Center became the first in Southeastern Wisconsin to use Intensity Modulated Radiation Therapy (IMRT), offering an unprecedented level of precision in radiation treatment. This was followed by a series of firsts and advanced technology for cancer treatment. Doctors began using radiofrequency ablation treatment to destroy tumors within the liver, kidney, and lungs. In 2002, Gliasite Radiation Therapy was added to deliver radiation directly to the site of the cancer, resulting in shorter treatments and fewer side effects.

That year also saw the introduction of real-time, four-dimensional ultrasound technology. Medical College surgeons at Froedtert were among the first in the country to use Gamma Knife radiosurgery that uses radiation to perform noninvasive brain surgery. As a result of the hospital's partnership with GE Healthcare, the world's first LightSpeed VCT, a revolutionary new CT scanner, was installed in 2004. That same year ushered in the TomoTherapy Hi-Art System that uses radiation to reach irregularly shaped tumors near critical organs and chemoembolization that delivers chemotherapy directly into the liver's blood supply. Other advances include: TheraSphere for patients with inoperable liver cancer, nerve-sparing surgery for prostate and testicular cancers, and High-Dose Brachytherapy to deliver concentrated radiation pellets to lumpectomy sites.

The hospital's national reputation continued to grow with multiple awards and special designations granted over the years:

- By 1997, Froedtert & the Medical College Cancer Center had been designated a "Teaching Hospital Cancer Program" by the Commission on Cancer of the American College of Surgeons.

- In 2000, *U.S. News and World Report* named Froedtert one of America's best hospitals for its departments of Kidney Disease, Digestive Disorders, and Orthopaedics.

- In 2002, *U.S. News and World Report* again named the hospital as one of the best, this time for its departments of Urology, Hormonal/Endocrine Disorders, and Kidney Disease.

- That same year, the American Association of Retired Persons' *Modern Maturity* named Froedtert Hospital one of the ten best in the nation for renal care.

The awards and recognition have continued:

- In 2005, the hospital's Palliative Care Program received the American Hospital Association's Circle of Life Award as one of the top ten in the nation.
- *Milwaukee Magazine* named Froedtert as one of the best places to work in 2005.
- In November 2006, Froedtert Hospital achieved Magnet designation for excellence in nursing services by the American Nurses Credential Center's Magnet Recognition Program®.
- More than 150 Medical College doctors practicing at Froedtert were recognized in the 2006 and 2007 listings of Best Doctors in America. No other hospital in Wisconsin lists more than Froedtert.
- The National Research Corporation bestowed a Consumer Choice Award on Froedtert in 2007, the fifth time the hospital was recognized. This nationwide survey asked more than 400,000 consumers to choose hospitals with the "best overall quality and image."
- Froedtert Hospital was selected as a "Best of Wisconsin Business" by *Corporate Report Wisconsin* and "Best Places to Work" by the *Business Journal* in 2006 and 2007.
- In 2007, *U.S. News and World Report* again listed Froedtert as one of "America's Best Hospitals" in the areas of Endocrinology, Kidney Disease, and Urology. Of 5,462 hospitals evaluated nationwide, only 173 qualified for the "Best Hospitals" list.

Recent professional recognition includes:

- The American College of Radiology accredited Froedtert's radiation oncology physicians; only 10 percent are accredited nationwide.
- The Comprehensive Rehabilitation, Brain Injury Rehabilitation, and Spinal Cord Injury programs at Froedtert are the only organizations in Wisconsin to hold Commission on Accreditation of Rehabilitation Facilities (CARF) accreditation in all three areas.
- The trauma center at Froedtert & the Medical College was reverified as a Level I Trauma Center by the Committee on Trauma of the American College of Surgeons in 2007.
- The Cancer Center's Blood and Marrow Transplant Program is one of only two in the state accredited by the Foundation for the Accreditation of Cellular Therapy.
- Froedtert & the Medical College recently received the American Stroke Association's Get with the Guidelines-Stroke Annual Performance Achievement Award. The award recognizes commitment and success in implementing a higher standard of stroke care.

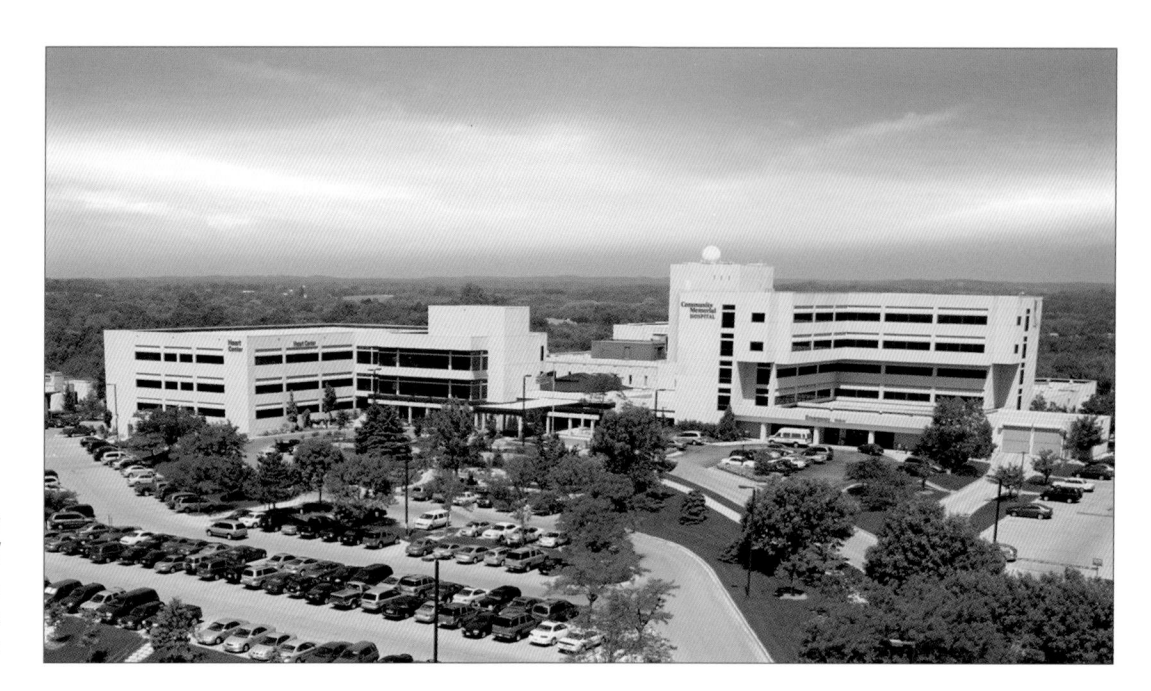

Community Memorial Hospital, Menomonee Falls, Wisconsin

Business achievements over those years were equally powerful. Among the highlights is Froedtert's leadership in the successful development of a community-based network for GA-MP that Milwaukee County, under the leadership of Paula Lucey, expanded to include primary care clinics throughout Milwaukee County and the participation of every hospital. The process also began to shift the care for all uninsured patients in a more equally distributed manner, and the network became a national model.

The dissolution of Horizon Healthcare resulted in the emergence of Froedtert & Community Health, a joining of Froedtert Hospital with Community Memorial Hospital of Menomonee Falls in a partnership committed to strengthening both organizations while retaining each hospital's strong identity and program. Other collaborative local and regional partnerships grew to include United Healthcare in Kenosha, ThedaCare in the Fox Valley, and Agnesian Healthcare in Fond du Lac.

Froedtert has maintained a consistent position among the highest achievers for quality of care and safety of environment as judged by the Joint Commission that accredits healthcare organizations. It developed a successful cost containment effort that shifted Froedtert from the most costly provider to the lowest average charge in metro Milwaukee by 2001, and today its charges are 12 percent below the market average. The focus on quality improvement has garnered national recognition for its application of the Six Sigma manufacturing error reduction methodology of medical errors. Froedtert & the Medical College are

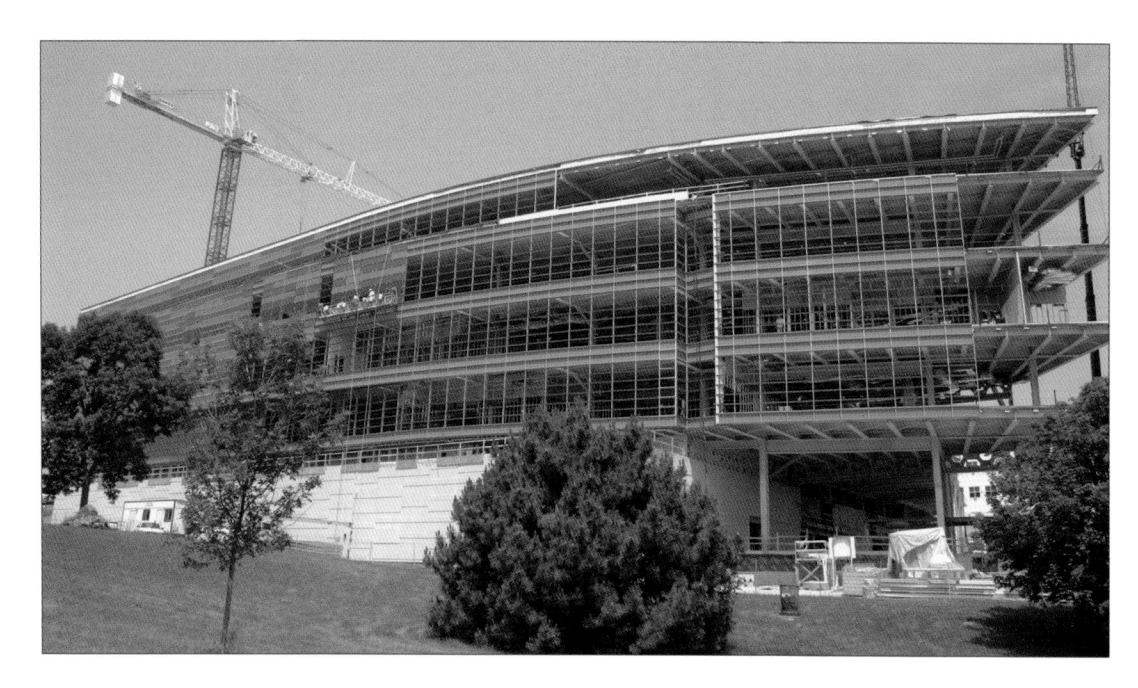

The whirlwind continues with the construction of the new Clinical Cancer Center.

founding members of the Collaborative for Healthcare Quality, a consortium of healthcare organizations working together to improve the quality of care in Wisconsin.

Froedtert Hospital has received national recognition for implementation of its construction philosophy of "logical not lavish." This philosophy is part of Froedtert's commitment to cost-efficient operations. The premise is to provide an attractive care environment without adding unnecessary costs to the process in terms of room size, amenities, and decorations. Froedtert also utilizes a conservative approach to new construction that is based on need. For example, on the inpatient side, new construction is based on occupancy, reaching 85 percent versus the general design standards of 70–74 percent occupancy. Under this conservative

Froedtert Hospital Leadership

Chairmen of the Froedtert Board of Directors

1980	William Jahn
1981-1983	Robert Foote
1984	I. Andrew Rader
1985-2000	Thomas L. Smallwood
2001-present	P. Michael Mahoney

Presidents and CEOs of Froedtert

1980-1993	Dean K. Roe
1993-present	William D. Petasnick

Milwaukee Regional Medical Center

BloodCenter of Wisconsin

Children's Hospital of Wisconsin

Curative Care Network

Froedtert Hospital

Medical College of Wisconsin

Milwaukee County Behavioral Health Division

> **Froedtert Memorial Lutheran Hospital**
>
> ### 2007 Board of Directors
>
> P. Michael Mahoney, Chairman
> Edward J. Zore, Vice Chairman
> William D. Petasnick, President and CEO
> David J. Lubar, Secretary
> Roger D. Peirce, Treasurer
>
> Kurt D. Bechthold
> Mary C. Cannon
> Curt S. Culver
> Edmund H. Duthie, Jr., MD
> William C. Hansen
> Geneva B. Johnson
> Dennis J. Kuester
> David N. Larson
> Pamela A. Maxson-Cooper,
>   Chief Nursing Officer
> Andrew J. Norton, MD
>   Chief Medical Officer
> Joan M. Prince, PhD
> Dennis J. Purtell
> John J. Stollenwerk
> Michael H. White
>
> *Director Emeritus:*
> Thomas A. Rosenberg (deceased)
>
> ### Froedtert Hospital Trust Trustees
>
> Robert B. Bradley
> Richard S. Gallagher
> John H. Hendee, Jr.
> Thomas F. Schrader

approach, Froedtert has still maintained a steady building program over the last twenty-five years. Additions have included: the East Clinics and Cancer Center, which opened in 1998; the five-story North Tower inpatient addition, which opened in 2002; and the freestanding Sargeant Health Center that houses outpatient clinics and surgery, which opened in 2005. Also in 2005, the old East Parking structure was demolished to make room for the new Clinical Cancer Center that is slated to open spring 2008. Another addition to the North Tower will open in 2009.

By the close of 2005, which marked the twenty-fifth anniversary of the opening of Froedtert Hospital, the vision of Kurtis Froedtert had been achieved. Froedtert had emerged as one of only 115 elite hospitals across the country designated as Academic Medical Centers. In partnership with the Medical College, Froedtert Hospital had become a community of learning at the forefront of medical care. This partnership has created a nationally recognized academic medical center that defines exceptional patient care, advances in technology, scientific discovery, and healthcare innovation. It is a hospital that brings unmatched resources and benefits to the greater Milwaukee community and Southeastern Wisconsin. After what has been deemed an incredible journey, today Froedtert Hospital is an extraordinary academic medical center. Kurtis Froedtert would be justifiably proud. ■

About the Author

The author of this book, James F. King, spent most of his career in the field of healthcare and most of his life on the grounds of what would become the Milwaukee Regional Medical Center. His father, Joseph King, MD, was director of surgery at Milwaukee County General Hospital for thirty-four years and one of the driving forces behind the creation of this academic medical center. Jim became the director of public information and marketing at Froedtert Hospital prior to its opening.

After graduating from Marquette University with a degree in journalism, Jim worked for thirteen years as a general news and sports reporter. He left the sports field to become director of public information and development at the Marquette University School of Medicine and later served as the public relations director at St. Joseph Hospital in Milwaukee. He and Karl Glunz established a consulting firm that provided long-range planning, communication, and marketing services to hospitals nationwide. Jim joined the Froedtert staff in 1980 and headed up the hospital's communications efforts until his retirement in 1995.

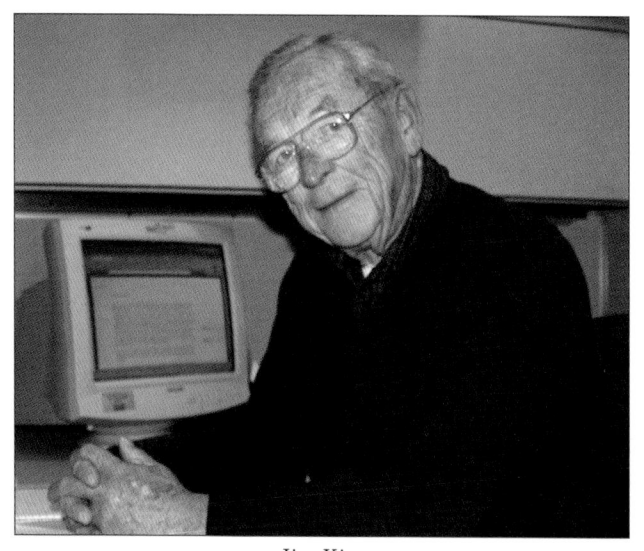

Jim King

Index

Page numbers in italics refer to photos.

Abert, Donald, 38
Accreditation Committee (Association of American Medical Colleges), 49
Adams, Dr. Mark, 120–21
Agnesian Healthcare (Fond du Lac), 126, 142
Alexander, Leonard, *44*
Allen-Bradley Medical Science laboratory (Milwaukee), 16
Ambulatory Care Agreement, 76
Ament, F. Thomas, 124, 128, 130, 131
American Association of Retired Persons, 141
American College of Radiology, 141
American College of Surgeons, 141
American Hospital Association, 126
 Circle of Life Award, 141
American Nurses Credentialing Center, 141
American Stroke Association, 141
Andreano, Ralph, 86–89, 92
Auxiliary. *See* Volunteer Associates, *114*, 114

Bachhuber, Dr. Edward, *44*
Baker, Robert J., 131
Baldwin, Susan, 123–24
Balzer, John, 112
Barron, Michael, 57
Bechthold, Kurt D., 144
beer/brewing industry, 3–4
Behrens, Elmer, 30, *67*

Bellin Health (Green Bay), 126
Benz, James, *93*, 93–94
Best Doctors in America list, 141
Bickel, Clarence, 30
Black Health Coalition, 124
Blatz Brewing Company, 9
BloodCenter of Wisconsin. *(*Blood Center of Wisconsin and Milwaukee Blood Center), 43, 45, 65, 75, 76, 123, 126, 143
Blue Ribbon study, 124
Blue Ribbon Task Force, 43
Board of Administration for Health and Social Services, 13
Bolger, T. Michael, 75, 128
Bradley, Robert, 66–68, 144
Brain Injury Rehabilitation Program, 141
brewing industry, 3–4
Bridge Building (Milwaukee Regional Medical Center), *69*, 69, 90–91, 101, 104
Brophy, Thomas, 130, 131–32, 134–35
Brunau, Joyce, 102
Brust-Zimmerman, 94
Buck, Cathy, 112
Bugbee, B. C., 18
Burroughs computer system, 117
Burroughs Corporation, 97–98
Business Journal, 124, 139, 141
Buss, Waldo, 18

Cannon, Mary C., 144
CARF (Commission on Accreditation of Rehabilitation Facilities), 141
Carley, David, 51, 78, 89, 91, 100
Carpenter, O. W., 38
Casey, Daniel, 124
Casey, Mr., 9
CAT scanner controversy, 102–4, *104*
Centers of Excellence, 134
Children's Hospital of Wisconsin (Milwaukee)
　classification, 79–80
　and Deaconess Hospital, 90
　and the Douglass Report, 123
　and the Medical College of Wisconsin, 134
　and the Milwaukee Regional Medical Center, 43, 45, 115, 116, 145
CHPASEW (Comprehensive Health Planning Agency of Southeastern Wisconsin), 25, 58, 79–80
Christbaum and Kehrein Brewery (Milwaukee), 3
Citizen's Governmental Research Bureau, 100
Cleary, Catherine, 18
Clinical Cancer Center (Milwaukee), *143*, 144
Clinical Research Laboratory (Milwaukee), 119
Coffey, William, 13, *13*
Coggs-Jones, Elizabeth, 124
College of Physicians and Surgeons (Milwaukee), 13, 14. See also Medical College of Wisconsin; Milwaukee County General Hospital
Collentine, Dr. George, *44*
Columbia Hospital (Milwaukee), 58, 129

Commission on Accreditation of Rehabilitation Facilities (CARF), 141
Commission on Cancer of the American College of Surgeons, 140
Community Memorial Hospital (Menomonee Falls), 126, 129, 142, *142*
Community Welfare Council, 38
Comprehensive Health Planning Act (1966), 56, 58–59, 69
Comprehensive Health Planning Agency of Southeastern Wisconsin (CHPASEW), 25, 58, 79–80
Comprehensive Rehabilitation Program, 141
Consumer Choice Award, 141
Cook, Dr. Harold E., 39, 45
Corporate Report Wisconsin, 141
cost-sharing ordinance (1973), 71–72
County Grounds. *See* Milwaukee County Institutions
Cowee, John, *44*
Cronkhite, Dr. Leonard W., Jr., 91
CT scanners, 140
Culver, Curt S., 144
Curative Care Network (Milwaukee), 43, 145
Curative Rehabilitation Center (Milwaukee), 123
Curative Workshop (Milwaukee), 61, 62, 63, 75

Davis, Jackie (*née* Schaeffer), *111*
Deaconess Hospital (Milwaukee), 47, 84–92, 97–98, 113, 115–16
　and the Children's Hospital of Wisconsin, 90
DeBakey, Dr. Michael, 38
DeBruin, Lynne, 130

DeCosse, Dr. Jerry, 109–10
Diagnosis Related Groups (DRGs), 118
Douglass (Robert) Associates, 122
Douglass Report, 122–23, 128, 129
Doyne, John, 37
    and the County Board, 56
    election to office, 25
    and the Froedtert Memorial Lutheran
        Hospital lease signing, 67
    and the Heil Report, 42–46
    and the Medical Center Steering
        Committee, 44
    and the Medical College of Wisconsin,
        70
    and the Medical College of Wisconsin
        lease signing, 77
    and the Milwaukee County Board, 124
    and the Milwaukee County General
        Hospital, 28
    and the Milwaukee County Institutions
        Grounds, 37–39
    and the Milwaukee Regional Medical
        Center, 58–60, 75
    and the Texas Medical Center, 35
    and Vogt, 32
Drew, William, 130
Dreyfus, Lee Sherman, 113, *113*
DRGs (Diagnosis Related Groups), 118
Duthie, Dr. Edmund H., Jr., 144
Dysphagia Institute, 120

economic effects of German immigration,
    3–4
Ellison, Dr. Edwin, 27
Ells, Ralph, 30
Elmbrook Hospital (Brookfield), 58
emergency care, 28, 110

Engstrom, Dr. William, 27
Evergreen Hospital (Seattle), 109
Eye Institute (Milwaukee), 70

Facility Planning and Development, 112
Fairchild, Thomas, 18
Falk, Harold F., 30
Fichtner, Pauline, 114
Findorff-Hutter, 96
Firmin, D. C., 35, 39
Fitzgerald, Edmund, 32, 34–35, *35*, 39, 43,
    44, 45
Fleming, Robert, 47
Foley, Leon F., 9, 18, 20, 22
Foley & Lardner, 9
Foote, Robert, 38, 143
Foster, Chester, 30
Foundation for the Accreditation of Cellular
    Therapy, 141
Foundation Hospital in Milwaukee, 116
Francis D. Murphy Medical Library
    (Milwaukee), 15
Frank, Mrs. Arthur, 18
Frederickson, Arvid, 30
free flap surgery, 120
Froedtert, Jacob, 4
Froedtert, Kurtis R., vii, 6, *8*
    charity of, 6–7, 8
    death of, 8
    father of, 4
    legal will, 7, 18–20, 29, 31, 66, 76
    life of, 4–7
    vision, vii, 3, 47–48, 88, 144
Froedtert, Mary, vii, 93, *93*, 113
Froedtert, William, 4, 4–5
Froedtert & Community Health
    (Milwaukee), 126, 142

Froedtert & the Medical College of
    Wisconsin (Milwaukee)
  Blood and Marrow Transplant
      Program, 141
  Cancer Center, 140, 141, 144
  Hand Center, 119
  Trauma Center, 141
Froedtert Brothers Commission Company, 4
Froedtert Grain and Malting Company,
    4–5, *5*
Froedtert Hospital Auxiliary, 114, *114*
Froedtert Hospital Board of Directors, 21,
    30, 33, 46, 47, 58, 66, 82, 113
Froedtert Memorial Lutheran Hospital
    (Milwaukee)
  additions, 142–43
  application/approval to build, 81–92, *88*
  and the Bridge Building, 69, *69*, 90–91,
      101, 104
  building structure, *54-54*, 94–96, *95*, 105,
      138
  CAT scanner controversy, 102–4, *104*
  and Community Memorial
      Hospital, 126, 141, *142*
  merger with Lutheran Hospital of
      Milwaukee, 84, 86–92, 97–98
  establishment, 3
  funding/finances, 21–22, 63–64, 66, 91,
      92, 117–24
  groundbreaking, vii, *93*, 93–96
  lease signing, 66–68, *67*, 76–78, *77*
  location, 17–20, 25–29, 47, 66, 68–69,
      94
  and Milwaukee County General Hospital's
      closing, 126–35, *133*
  and the Milwaukee Regional Medical
      Center, 43, 66–69, 75–78, 81, 144

  opening day, *113*, 113–14
  planning, 11–16, 17–20, 25–29, 30–33,
      41–46
  reputation, 119–22, 139–43
  services, 110
  staff, 102, 105, 109–12, *111*, 125–27
  vs. the Comprehensive Health Planning
      Agency of Southeastern Wisconsin,
      79–80
Froedtert Memorial Lutheran Hospital
    Trust, 7, 8–9, 15–16, 17–20, 46, 66,
    89
Froedtert trustees, 8–9, 10, 21–22, 30–31
Fuchs, Margaret, 102
Fuller, Howard, 123

Gallagher, Richard S., 144
Gamma Knife radiosurgery, 140
GA-MP (General Assistance-Medical
    Program), 132, 133, 135, 142
gastroenterology, 120
GE Medical Systems, 119, 139, 140
General Assistance-Medical Program
    (GA-MP), 132, 133, 135, 142
General Clinical Research Center
    (Milwaukee), 120
German English Academy (Milwaukee), 5
German immigration's economic effects, 3–4
Gliasite Radiation Therapy, 140
GMC. *See* Greater Milwaukee Committee
Good Samaritan Medical Center
    (Milwaukee), 115–16
Gottlieb, Symond, 32, 41, *44*
Graduate School of Biomedical Sciences
    (Milwaukee), 134
Greater Milwaukee Committee (GMC)
  and Doyne, 39

and the Froedtert Hospital Corporation, 31
and Froedtert Memorial Lutheran
Hospital, 115
and the Heil Report, vii
and the Hospital Area Planning
Committee, 41–46
and the McLean Report, 15–16
and the Medical College of Wisconsin,
58
and medical school funding, 50
and the Milwaukee County Medical
Complex, 124
role, 34–36
Grede, Arthur L., 30

Hamilton (James A.) and Associates, 28, 33,
47, 89
Hand Center. *See* Froedtert & the Medical
College of Wisconsin Hand Center,
119
Hansen, Terrence M., 128–29, 130
Hansen, William C., 144
Hanser, Mary Julia (Julie), 123, 125,
127
Hantke Brewing School, 5
HAPC (Hospital Area Planning Committee),
31, 34–35, 41–46, 58
Heil, Joseph, 39–40, 43, *44*, 50
Heil Report (Greater Milwaukee Committee),
vii, 43–44, 45–46
Hendee, John H., Jr., 144
Henderson, Bernice, 114
Henderson, Bob, 114
Hering, Carla, 114, *114*
Herriott, Maxwell, 66
High-Dose Brachytherapy, 140
Hill-Burton, 21

Hirschboeck, Dr. John
and Doyne, 38–39
and the Heil Report, 43, *43*
and medical school funding, 9, 14–15, 49
and the Milwaukee Regional Medical
Center, 33
and the Milwaukee Sanitarium, 18, 20
and the Texas Medical Center, 35
and the University Medical Center
Corporation of Milwaukee, 22
and the Veteran's Administration Hospital,
28
Holloway, Lee, 129–31
Horizon Healthcare, Inc., 129, 142
Hospital Area Planning Committee (HAPC),
31, 34–35, 41–46, 58
Hyatt and Associates, 99–100

immigration's economic effects, 3–4
IMRT (Intensity Modulated Radiation
Therapy), 140
Intensity Modulated Radiation Therapy
(IMRT), 140
Interim Guidance Committee, 115

Jackson, Robert, 124, 128–31
Jacobus, Delbert C., 39, *44*, 45, 67
Jahn, William, 30, 67, 68, 77, 93, 93–94,
143
Jamron, Ken, 87, 97
Janssen, William, 9
Jenkins, William I., 123
John L. Doyne Hospital (Milwaukee), 125,
127–35, *133*. *See also* Milwaukee
County General Hospital
Johnson, Geneva B., 144
Johnson, Lyndon, 38–39

Joint Commission on the Accreditation of Healthcare Organizations, 142
Joint Finance Committee, 50
Joint Management Committee, 123
Joint Medical Computer Services Center (Milwaukee), 97–98
Junkerman, Dr. Carl, *108*, 109–10

Kelley, James, 38
Kerrigan, Dr. Gerald, 35, 38, 39, *44*, 45, 50, 74, 75
Keyes, James, 128–29
Kincaid, Douglas, 33
King, Jim, vii, 145, *145*
King, Dr. Joseph M., 13–14, 16, *16*
Klag, E. D., *44*
Klotsche, Dr. J. Martin, 30, 39, *44*
Knowles, Warren, 50
Kradwell, Dr. William, 18, 20
Krebs, Alice, 114
Krivitz, James, 100
Krumbiegel, Dr. Edward, *44*
Krzewinski, Elizabeth, 38, *44*
Kuester, Dennis J., 144
Kurtis R. Froedtert Memorial Lutheran Hospital Corporation, 30–33

Landis, Dr. Charles, *44*
Larson, Dr. David, 120, 144
Lartner, Mary, 109
Law, John T., 11
LCME (Licensing Committee for Medical Education), 22
Liaison Committee on Medical Education, 8–9
Licensing Committee for Medical Education (LCME), 22

Lindner, Fred, 38, 39, *44*
Logan, Edward, 35, 39, *44*
Lubar, David J., 144
Lucey, Patrick, 51
Lucey, Paula, 135, 142
Lutheran Hospital of Milwaukee, 21, 32, 47–48, 84, 86–92, 97–98, 113, 115–16
Lutheran Men in America of Wisconsin, 29, 30, 50
Lyons, Willard (Mike), 37

MACC Fund Research Center (Milwaukee), 134
Madison, Dr. Frederick W., 22
Mahoney, P. Michael, 143, 144
Marquette School of Medicine (Milwaukee), 29, 43, 50–51. *See also* Medical College of Wisconsin
Marquette University School of Medicine (Milwaukee), 7–10, 13–16, 21–22, 25, 31, 42–45, *49*, 49–51. *See also* Medical College of Wisconsin
Marquette University student health clinic (Milwaukee), 16
Matloub, Dr. Hani, 119
Maxson-Cooper, Pam, 112, 144
Mayfair Mall (Wauwatosa), 9–10, 17, *17*
McCarty, Dr. Daniel, 110
McFetridge, Georgiana, 22, 59
McLean, Dr. Basil, 11–15, 18
McLean Report, 12, 15–17, 25, 31, 39–40, 43, 45, 48
McNerney, Walter, 97
Medical Center Council, 71, 79
Medical Center of Southeastern Wisconsin (Milwaukee), 64

Medical College Basic Science building
(Milwaukee), 27, 45, 51, 61, 62, 70,
71, 74, 78, 91
Medical College Board, 89
Medical College Executive Committee,
75
Medical College of Wisconsin (Milwaukee).
See also College of Physicians and
Surgeons; Marquette School of
Medicine; Marquette University
School of Medicine
and the Children's Hospital of Wisconsin,
134
and the Douglass Report, 123
and Froedtert Memorial Lutheran
Hospital, vii, 89, 141, 143
funding, 9, 73–78
and the Greater Milwaukee Committee, 58
and the Heil Report, 43
lease signing, 70–72
and Milwaukee County General Hospital,
99–100
and the Milwaukee County Institutions
Grounds, 61–62
and the Milwaukee Regional Medical
Center, 145
public/private ownership, 49–51
reputation, 118–19, 139
software programs, 97–98
and the Veteran's Administration Hospital,
28
Medical College of Wisconsin Board, 125
Medical College of Wisconsin Hand
Center (Milwaukee), 119, *119*
Medical Society of Milwaukee County, 116
Medicare/Medicaid issues, 31–32, 38–39, 56,
81–82, 99, 118

Mental Health Center (Milwaukee), 89, 91,
100
Mental Health Complex (Milwaukee),
70
Metropolitan Milwaukee Association of
Commerce, 115
Milwaukee, 2
Milwaukee Arena, 34
Milwaukee Art Museum, 34
Milwaukee County Behavioral Health
Division, 43, 143
Milwaukee County Board
and the Bridge Building, 69
bureaucracy, 122
members, 56, 57–60
and Milwaukee County General Hospital,
132
and the Milwaukee Regional Medical
Center, 73
Milwaukee County Board Finance
Committee, 70, 91, 99, 131
Milwaukee County Board Health
Committee, 56, 57, 61–69, 70, 71,
73, 131
Milwaukee County Board of Public Welfare,
28, 31, 37, 55, 61, 73–75
Milwaukee County Board of Supervisors,
51, 56, 70, 130, 131
Milwaukee County Courthouse, 99
Milwaukee County Executive Budget,
122–23
Milwaukee County General Hospital. *See
also* Milwaukee County Medical
Complex
buildings, *12, 24–25*
and the Douglass Report, 122
finances, 99–101

Milwaukee County General Hospital
    (continued)
    and Froedtert Memorial Lutheran
        Hospital, 81–82, 89, 126–35
    funding, 79
    and the Heil Report, 45–46
    location, 68–69
    losses, 116–18
    Medicare/Medicaid issues, 32
    and the Milwaukee Regional Medical
        Center, 42, 51
    purchase of Doyne Hospital, *133*
    services, 110
    teaching programs, 12–15, 25–26
    and Veteran's Administration Hospital, 28
Milwaukee County government, 31, 42
Milwaukee County Institutions Grounds, *100*
    buildings, *11*
    facilities, 12–13, 37–38
    and Froedtert Memorial Lutheran
        Hospital, vii
    and the Milwaukee Regional Medical
        Center, 42, 45, 55–56, 59, 61, 63,
        71–74
Milwaukee County Medical Complex, *24-25*,
    122–24
Milwaukee County Medical Society, 62–63
Milwaukee County Services Board, 101
Milwaukee County Stadium, 34
Milwaukee County Zoo, 34
Milwaukee Journal
    on Doyne, 59
    on Froedtert, 5–7, 19–20
    on Froedtert Memorial Lutheran
        Hospital, 82
    on the Medical College of Wisconsin,
        64–65
    on the Milwaukee County Medical
        Complex, 124
    on the Milwaukee Regional Medical
        Center, 74, 100–101
    on the Milwaukee Regional Medical
        Center, 42, 62–63
Milwaukee Lutheran, 29
Milwaukee Magazine, 141
Milwaukee Medical Center Council, 57–58
Milwaukee Medical Center Steering
    Committee, *44*, 45, 57–58
Milwaukee Medical Center Study Committee,
    39
Milwaukee Psychiatric Hospital, 45, 115
Milwaukee Regional Medical Center
    (MRMC)
    and the Allen-Bradley Medical Science
        laboratory, 16
    and the Bridge Building, *69*
    and the Children's Hospital of Wisconsin,
        43, 45, 115
    and the Douglass Report, 122–23
    finances, 100–101
    and Froedtert Memorial Lutheran
        Hospital, 8, 81, 90–91
    funding, 73–80
    and the Greater Milwaukee Committee,
        35
    and the Heil Report, 43
    members, 145
    and the Milwaukee County Institutions
        Grounds, 55–56, 61–69
    staff, 125
Milwaukee Sanitarium (Wauwatosa), *17*,
    17–20, 25–26, 28, 33, 45, 115
Milwaukee Sanitarium Foundation, 18, 21,
    28

Milwaukee Sentinel, 18–19, 28, 35–36, 86–87, 124
Milwaukee *Small Business Times* Health Care Hero Award, 109
Milwaukee University School, 5
Misericordia Hospital (Milwaukee), 47, 58
Modern Maturity, 140
Monfried, Walter, 5–7
Mount Sinai Hospital (Milwaukee), 47, 115
MRMC. *See* Milwaukee Regional Medical Center
Mulcahy, Charles, 57, 65
Mundt, Donald, 84, 89–90
Murphy, Dr. Francis D., 13–14, *15*

National Institutes of Health (Bethesda), 63
National Research Corporation, 141
neurosurgery, 120, 139
Northwestern Mutual Life Insurance Company, 34, 35, 43. 84, 103
Norton, Dr. Andrew J., 144
Nowakowski, Richard, 57, 59, 74–75
Nuzum, John, 39

Ochsner, Dr. Alton, 47
O'Connell, Blaine, 130
O'Donnell, James, 67, 68, 75
O'Donnell, William J.
    and Froedtert Memorial Lutheran Hospital, *93*, 93–94
    and the Froedtert Memorial Lutheran Hospital lease signing, *67*
    and the Medical Center Steering Committee, *44*
    and the Medical College of Wisconsin lease signing, 77

and medical school funding, 9
and the Milwaukee County Institutions Grounds, 37–38
and the Milwaukee Regional Medical Center, 64, 100–101
and the Texas Medical Center, 35
Orchard Lake Military Academy, 5
Ordinans, Karen, 130–31
organ transplants, 120–21, *121*, 139–40
Orlich, Sam, 57
otolaryngology, 120
Ott, Howard T., 9

Paige, John H., 30
Palliative Care Program, 141
Patrinos, Dan, 35–36
Pease, Harry, 63, 64–65
Peirce, Roger D., 144
Petasnick, William D., vii, *114*, *129*
    administration, 102
    and Froedtert Memorial Lutheran Hospital, 125–29, *127*, *129*, 131–32, 139, 143, 144
    and Milwaukee County General Hospital, 130–32, *133*
    and Roe, *125*
    and Smallwood, *114*
Petersen, Dr. John R., *44*, 45, 127–29, 130
Phillips, Ernest, 67
Pitts, Terrance, 57, 61–62, 64–65, 67, 75, 85, 86, 124
plastic surgery, 120
Pratt, Paul, 18
Prince, Joan M., 144
Profit, Pat, *111*
public/private ownership, 49–51, 59–61
Purtell, Dennis J., 144

Purtell, Dr. Robert, 38, 39, *44*

Rader, I. Andrew, *44*, 143
radiology, 110, 139
Rapkin, Joseph E., 9, *9*, 19, 67, *93*, 93–94
Rattan, Dr. Walter, 79
Raynor, John, 49
reconstructive surgery, 120
Regional Medical Program legislation, 38–39
replant operations, 119
Riley, Donovan, 86
Roe, Dean K.
   administration, 102–3
   and the Froedtert Board of Directors, 48
   and Froedtert Memorial Lutheran Hospital, 82, 84, 87, 89–90, 94, 96–97, 143
   and the Froedtert Memorial Lutheran Hospital lease signing, *67*
   and Froedtert Memorial Lutheran Hospital's services, 110
   and hospital affiliates, 118
   and the Medical College of Wisconsin lease signing, 77, *77*–78
   and the Milwaukee County Medical Complex, *123*
   and the Milwaukee Regional Medical Center, 33, 58, 64
   and the Milwaukee Sanitarium, 28, 39
   and Petasnick, 125, *125*
   and the Texas Medical Center, 35
Roper, Wayne, 67, 68, 76, 102
Rosenbaum, Dr. Francis, *44*
Rosenberg, Thomas A., 144
Rosenfeld, Eugene, 51
Rourke (Anthony J. J.), Inc., 89

Runge, Charlie, 135
Russell, Robert, 75

Samaritan Hospital, 117
Sanger, Dr. James, 119
Sargeant, Dr. Harry W., 13–14, *14*
Sargeant Health Center (Milwaukee), 144
Schoenecker, Rudolph, *44*, 67
Schrader, Thomas F., 144
Schroeder, Mrs. Gerhard H., 18, 20
Schwingle, Clement, 94
Seidemann, William A., 30
Senelly, Sue, *111*
Seton Health Corporation of Wisconsin, 129
7-70 plan, 109
SEWHSA (Southeastern Wisconsin Health Systems Agency), 41, 82, 84–88, 115–16
Shaughnessy, William J., 76
Shepard, John R., 90
Sheridan, Michael, 19
shock wave therapy, 121
Siebert, Reginald L., 30, 67
Six Sigma methodology, 126, 142
Slichter, Donald, 39
Small Business Times, 109
Smallwood, Thomas L., *114*, 128–29, *129*, 145
Smith, Mary Alice, 114
Smith, Symuel, 99–100
Smith (Herman) Associates, 89
Southeastern Wisconsin Health Systems Agency (SEWHSA), 41, 82, 84–88, 115–16
Spinal Cord Injury Program, 141
St. Anthony Hospital, 116
St. Joseph's Hospital (Milwaukee), 58

St. Luke's Hospital (Milwaukee), 21, 32, 47, 58
St. Mary's Hill Hospital (Milwaukee), 129
St. Mary's Hospital (Milwaukee), 123, 129
St. Mary's–Ozaukee Hospital (Mequon), 129
Stanislawski, Emil, 99
State Division of Health Policy and Planning, 69, 81, 82, 86
State Investment Board, 78
Steelman, Julien R., 30
Stevenson, Robert, 50, 67
Stollenwerk, John J., 144
Stone, Maracini, and Patterson, 94
Sullivan, Dr. James, 38, 39, *44*

Task Force on Medical Education, 50
teaching/training programs, 12–14, 16, 46, 81, 118–19, 134, 144
Texas Medical Center (Houston), 35–36
ThedaCare (Fox Valley), 126, 142
TomoTherapy Hi-Art System, 140
transplant surgery, 120–21, *121*, 139–40

United HealthCare (Kenosha), 142
United Hospital System, 126
United Regional Medical Services, 110
University Medical Center Corporation of Milwaukee, 22, 35, *59*
University of Wisconsin (Milwaukee), 7, 10, 42, 48, 70, 126
University of Wisconsin Hospital (Madison), 79, 83, 126
urology, 120, 121
U.S. News and World Report, 140, 141

Valenti, John J., 64–65

Veterans Administration Hospital (Milwaukee), 27–29, 45, 71, 73, 94
Vogt, Richard E., *30*, 30–33, 67, *93*, 93–94
Volunteer Associates. See Auxiliary, *114*, 114
Von Kohn, Maggie, 114

War Memorial (Milwaukee), 34
Wauwatosa Common Council, 69
Wauwatosans for Tomorrow, 114
Wedemeyer, Ted, 38, *44*
Werwath, Karl O., 30
Westgate shopping center. *See also* Mayfair Mall, 9–10
White, Michael H., 144
Willard, Dr. William R., 25
Willard Report, 25, 31, 43, 45
Wilson, Carlton P., 42, 43
Wisconsin Collaborative for Healthcare Quality, 126, 143
Wisconsin Division of Health Policy and Planning, 56, 125
Wisconsin Memorial Park (Milwaukee), 9–10

Yousif, Dr. John, 119

Zablocki, Clement J., 27
Zablocki, Thomas, 67
Zablocki Veteran's Hospital (Milwaukee), 121
Zimmerman Architectural Studios (Milwaukee), 94
Zoller, Gerd, 96
Zore, Edward J., 144